Current Developments in the Detection and Control of Multi Drug Resistance

Edited by

Sanket Kaushik

Amity Institute of Biotechnology
Amity University Rajasthan
Jaipur- 303002,
India

&

Nagendra Singh

School of Biotechnology
Gautam Buddha University
Greater Noida- 201308,
India

Current Developments in the Detection and Control of Multi Drug Resistance

Editors: Sanket Kaushik and Nagendra Singh

ISBN (Online): 978-981-5049-87-9

ISBN (Print): 978-981-5049-88-6

ISBN (Paperback): 978-981-5049-89-3

© 2022, Bentham Books imprint.

Published by Bentham Science Publishers Pte. Ltd. Singapore. All Rights Reserved.

First published in 2022.

need for a court order if at any point you breach any terms of this License Agreement. In no event will any delay or failure by Bentham Science Publishers in enforcing your compliance with this License Agreement constitute a waiver of any of its rights.

3. You acknowledge that you have read this License Agreement, and agree to be bound by its terms and conditions. To the extent that any other terms and conditions presented on any website of Bentham Science Publishers conflict with, or are inconsistent with, the terms and conditions set out in this License Agreement, you acknowledge that the terms and conditions set out in this License Agreement shall prevail.

Bentham Science Publishers Pte. Ltd.
80 Robinson Road #02-00
Singapore 068898
Singapore
Email: subscriptions@benthamscience.net

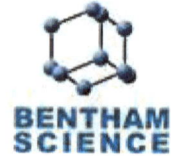

BENTHAM SCIENCE

CONTENTS

PREFACE

The ability of different species of bacteria to resist the antimicrobial agent has become a global problem. Despite the development of so many antibiotic molecules during the last fifty years, increasing antibiotic resistance worldwide may lead to therapeutic dead-end. The disease burden from multidrug-resistant strains of organisms causing AIDS, tuberculosis, gonorrhoea, malaria, influenza, pneumonia, and diarrhoea is being felt in both the developed and the developing countries alike. This book summarizes the emerging trends in the field of antibiotic resistance of various MDR bacterial species.

Current strategies of detection and control of multidrug resistant bacteria provides the clear and recent information regarding strategies involved in diagnosis and treatment of MDR bacteria. Over the past decades, due to the exponential rise in the infections caused by MDR bacteria, it is necessary to elucidate the basic mechanism of antibiotic resistance to find out the effective methods for treatment and control. Primary goal of this book is to elaborate and enhance the theoretical knowledge of bacterial pathogenesis, diagnosis and treatment. It concentrates on further elaboration of current strategies of detection and control of MDR bacteria, Quantification of pathogenic bacteria, High Resolution Melting Analysis techniques, Biosynthesis pathways and Rational structure based drug design for MDR infections.

We have attempted to provide large amount of information in each chapter supplemented with in- depth knowledge of current strategies of detection and control of MDR bacteria. This book enhances the knowledge of Microbiology, Biotechnology and Life sciences in field area of MDR pathogenesis and control. The idea to encompass knowledge spanning from what is known to what is unknown in the writings from the experts in the field will result in a rigorous effort to justify the various topics.

We strongly believe that this book will be reader's delight providing comprehensive understanding of diagnosis and treatment of MDR bacteria. It will be an ideal resource for student's better understanding of MDR bacteria biology and useful for biomedical students, cellular and molecular biologists. I hope you will find this book interesting and relevant.

Sanket Kaushik
Amity Institute of Biotechnology
Amity University Rajasthan
Jaipur- 303002, India

&

Nagendra Singh
School of Biotechnology
Gautam Buddha University
Greater Noida- 201308, India

List of Contributors

Aakanksha Kalra Dr B. Lal Institute of Biotechnology, Jaipur, 302017, India

Amit Alok Division of Radiation Biodosimetry, Institute of Nuclear Medicine and Allied Sciences, Timarpur, Delhi, 110054, India

Anupam Jyoti Department of Biotechnology, University Institute of aBiotechnology, Chandigarh University, Mohali, Punjab, 140413, India

Anurag Jyoti Amity University Madhya Pradesh, Maharajpura Dang, Gwalior-474005, M.P., India

Ayushi Khurana School of Biotechnology, Gautam Buddha University, Greater Noida, India

Divyapriya Karthikeyan Centre for Bioseparation Technology (CBST), Vellore Institute of Technology (VIT), Vellore, Tamil Nadu, India

Ena Gupta Amity Institute of Biotechnology, Amity University Rajasthan, Amity Education Valley, Kant Kalwar, NH-11C, Jaipur-Delhi Highway, Jaipur, India

Gunjan Shaily School of Biotechnology, Gautam Buddha University, Greater Noida, India

Juhi Saxena Department of Biotechnology, University Institute of aBiotechnology, Chandigarh University, Mohali, Punjab, 140413, India

Jyoti Yadav Amity Institute of Biotechnology, Amity University Rajasthan, Jaipur-303002, India

Kali Kishore Reddy Tetala Centre for Bio Separation Technology (CBST), Vellore Institute of Technology, Vellore, Tamil Nadu, India

Kishore K.R. Tetala Centre for Bioseparation Technology (CBST), Vellore Institute of Technology (VIT), Vellore, 632014, Tamil Nadu, India

Kumar Sambhav Verma Amity Institute of Biotechnology, Amity University Rajasthan, NH 11 C Kant Kalwar, Jaipur, India

Monish Bisen Faculty of Applied Sciences and Biotechnology, Shoolini University of Biotechnology and Management Sciences, Bajhol, Solan, Himachal Pradesh 173229, India

Mrinalini Roy Amity Institute of Biotechnology, Amity University Rajasthan, Kant Kalwar, NH-11C, Jaipur-Delhi Highway, Jaipur, India

Mukesh Kumar Department of Biophysics, All India Institute of Medical Sciences, New Delhi, New Delhi, India

Nagendra Singh School of Biotechnology, Gautam Buddha University, Greater Noida- 201308, India

Priyal Sharma Amity Institute of Biotechnology, Amity University Rajasthan, NH 11 C Kant Kalwar, Jaipur, India

Punit Kaur Department of Biophysics, All India Institute of Medical Sciences, New-Delhi, India

Rajesh Singh Tomar Amity Institute of Biotechnology, Amity University Madhya Pradesh, Maharajpura Dang, Gwalior-474005, M.P., India

Ravi Ranjan Kumar Niraj	Amity Institute of Biotechnology, Amity University Rajasthan, Jaipur, 303002, India
Ravneet Chug	Amity Institute of Biotechnology, Amity University Rajasthan, NH 11 C Kant Kalwar, Jaipur, India
Sakshi Piplani	Vaxine Pty Ltd, Warradale, Australia; College of Medicine and Public Health, Flinders University, Adelaide, Australia
Sanjit Kumar	Centre for Bioseparation Technology (CBST), Vellore Institute of Technology (VIT), Vellore, Tamil Nadu, India
Sanket Kaushik	Amity Institute of Biotechnology, Amity University Rajasthan, Jaipur- 303002, India
Sudhir Kumar Pal	Centre for Bio Separation Technology (CBST), Vellore Institute of Technology, Vellore, Tamil Nadu, India
Vaishali Gurjar	School of Biotechnology, Gautam Buddha University, Greater Noida, India
Vijay Kumar Srivastava	Amity Institute of Biotechnology, Amity University Rajasthan, Amity Education Valley, Kant Kalwar, NH-11C, Jaipur-Delhi Highway, Jaipur, India
Vijay Pal	Amity Institute of Biotechnology, Amity University Rajasthan, NH 11 C Kant Kalwar, Jaipur, India
Vinay Sharma	Amity Institute of Biotechnology, Amity University Rajasthan, Jaipur-303002, India
Vinod Singh Gour	Amity Institute of Biotechnology, Amity University Rajasthan, NH 11 C Kant Kalwar, Jaipur, India

CHAPTER 1

Introduction

Sanket Kaushik[1] and Nagendra Singh[2,*]

[1] *Amity Institute of Biotechnology, Amity University Rajasthan, Jaipur- 303002, India*

[2] *School of Biotechnology, Gautam Buddha University, Greater Noida- 201308, India*

Antimicrobial resistance occurs naturally over time due to changes at the genetic level of microorganisms. These microorganisms are present in food, animals, plants, humans, and the environment. Many pathogens can spread from people to people or from animals to humans. Some of the major drivers of the development of antimicrobial resistance are misuse (overuse, inappropriate selection and/or dosing, *etc.*) of antimicrobial agents, poor infection and disease management, lack of access to clean water, sanitation and hygiene for the people, poor access to affordable and quality drugs and diagnostics, lack of awareness and knowledge about health care, *etc*.

The global resistance among various pathogenic microbes to antimicrobial drugs is now becoming a serious threat to public health worldwide. The failure of treating microbial diseases is leading to prolonged illness and higher expenditure on healthcare along with a greater risk of life. Today, most infectious agents, including viruses, bacteria, fungi and parasites, have developed Multi-Drug Resistance (MDR), which is responsible for drastic increase in morbidity and mortality. In the last few decades, the administration of antibiotics has drastically increased due to a rapid rate of microbial infections; the latter owed to the emergence of MDR in various microbial strains. MDR is defined as a reduced sensitivity of a microbe to an antimicrobial drug that had been used effectively against the same microbe earlier. Such resistant organisms are able to combat the drug leading to ineffective treatment and increased persistence and spreading of the infection in an individual or population.

Antibiotics are a class of chemotherapeutic agents used in the clinical management of microbial infections. Although antibiotics have been used as magic bullets for curing various bacterial infections, their benefits are diminished due to the global emergence of resistant bacterial strains. The term antibiotics was

---

[*] **Corresponding author Nagendra Singh:** School of Biotechnology, Gautam Buddha University, Greater Noida-201308, India; E-mail: nagendratomar@gmail.com

first coined by Selman Walksman, an American microbiologist, for compounds that inhibit the growth of microorganisms [1]. The modern era of antibiotics started in 1928 with the discovery of penicillin from the culture of the fungus *Penicillium notatum* by Alexander Fleming, a British doctor. Although the development of antibiotic resistance is mainly attributed to the imprudent and excessive usage of antibiotics, both biosynthetic antibiotic as well as resistance-conferring genes have been known to have evolved much before the use of antibiotics [2 - 5]. The natural occurrence of antibiotics in sub- inhibitory amounts acts as signaling molecules for quorum sensing, biofilm formation, and in production of virulence factors. The elucidation of the precise roles and mechanisms of antibiotics still remains to be understood. Antibiotics are secondary metabolites of microorganisms that are produced in a very low concentration during the late stages of the stationary growth phase. The drastically different roles of antibiotics have been explored in natural conditions in comparison to the high doses used for therapeutic purposes against microbes. Nutrient starvation induces microbes to produce a large array of small compounds called parvomes [6]. So far, only a small fraction of parvomes has been characterized as antimicrobial agents.

WHO has reported rapid MDR emergence in *E. coli, K. pneumonia, S. pneumonia, Mycobacterium tuberculosis* and species of *Salmonella* and *Shigella* spp. for a number of antibiotic molecules [7]. Various fungi such as *Candida, Aspergillus* spp., *Cryptococcus neoformans, Trichosporon beigelii, Scopulariopsis* spp., and *Pseudallescheria boydii* have been reported as resistant against drugs such as polyene macrolides, azole derivatives, nucleotide synthesis inhibitors and 1,3-β-glucan synthase inhibitors [7, 8]. An extended exposure to antiviral drugs has made viruses also resistant in immunocompromised people. MDR has been observed in several viruses such as cytomegalovirus (CMV), herpes simplex (HSV), Varicella-Zoster (VZV), human immunodeficiency (HIV), influenza A, hepatitis C (HCV), and hepatitis B (HBV) viruses [9, 10]. MDR emergence has also been reported in several parasites, including *Plasmodium spp., Leishmania spp., Entamoeba spp., Trichomonas vaginalis, Schistosoma* spp. and *Toxoplasma gondii* for drugs such as pentavalent antimonials, miltefosine, chloroquine, artemisinin, paromomycin, amphotericin B, atovaquone, sulfadiazine and pyrimethamine [11 - 19].

Most of the infectious organisms have developed high level of alarming MDR against many commonly used antibiotics, being called "super bugs". Examples of super bugs include MDR bacteria causing urinary tract infections, skin infections and pneumonia. Resistance is known to be a naturally occurring process. A lot of research is currently being performed in order to gain better understanding of resistance mechanisms, which will further aid in tackling the resistant microbes.

The emergence of MDR is a serious threat to society in the current era, since influenza, HIV, tuberculosis, pneumonia, yeast infections and other diseases are major causes of mortality. As per the WHO's update, in 2018, 3.5% new cases and 18% old cases of tuberculosis in the world are estimated to present MDR. About 8.5% of MDR cases showed extensive drug resistance (XDR) tuberculosis. Over 40,000 cases of XDR-TB cases are projected to be emerging every year. MDR-TB is caused by bacteria that do not respond to at least two of the most potent drugs, isoniazid and rifampicin. Pneumonia is one of the most common infections globally. MDR Gram negative bacteria (MDR-GNB) are responsible for serious threats to the health care system. The most common *Enterobacteriaceae* isolated from patients with pneumonia were found to be *Klebsiella pneumoniae*, *Enterobacter* spp. and *Escherichia coli*, which accounted for 12%, 8%, and 7%, respectively, of all bacterial isolates included in a study [20]. Antiretroviral therapy for HIV also faces severe challenges due to the development of resistance. Similarly, malaria parasites have also been observed to be resistant to several drugs such as chloroquine, artemisinin, and pyrimethamine [18].

In recent times, infections by MDR microbes have become a big issue in public healthcare management. The overuse or misuse of antibiotic agents in the last few decades is responsible for the emergence of several MDR strains of bacteria, viruses, fungi and parasites. A rapid increase of severe systemic infections along with the development and spread of resistant pathogens are creating a serious challenge to the current healthcare system. Regrettably, so far, the efforts to develop new drugs have not been sufficient to tackle the emergence of new MDR strains. Along with implementing social awareness programs, there is an urgent need to understand the development of resistance mechanisms to find a therapeutic solution for the MDR microorganisms.

CONSENT FOR PUBLICATION

Not applicable.

CONFLICT OF INTEREST

The authors declare no conflict of interest, financial or otherwise.

ACKNOWLEDGEMENTS

Declared none.

REFERENCES

[1]   Waksman SA. The role of antibiotics in nature. Perspect Biol Med 1961; 4(3): 271-87.
        [http://dx.doi.org/10.1353/pbm.1961.0001]

[2]   Tanwar J, Das S, Fatima Z, Hameed S. Multidrug resistance: an emerging crisis. Interdiscip Perspect Infect Dis 2014; 2014: 541340.
        [http://dx.doi.org/10.1155/2014/541340] [PMID: 25140175]

[3]   Gullberg E, Cao S, Berg OG, *et al.* Selection of resistant bacteria at very low antibiotic concentrations. PLoS Pathog 2011; 7(7): e1002158.
        [http://dx.doi.org/10.1371/journal.ppat.1002158] [PMID: 21811410]

[4]   Davies J. Darwin and microbiomes. EMBO Rep 2009; 10(8): 805.
        [http://dx.doi.org/10.1038/embor.2009.166] [PMID: 19648955]

[5]   Fleming A. Classics in infectious diseases: on the antibacterial action of cultures of a *penicillium,* with special reference to their use in the isolation of *B. influenzae* by Alexander Fleming, Reprinted from the British Journal of Experimental Pathology 10:226-236, 1929. Rev Infect Dis 1980; 2(1): 129-39.
        [http://dx.doi.org/10.1093/clinids/2.1.129] [PMID: 6994200]

[6]   Sengupta S, Chattopadhyay MK, Grossart H-P. The multifaceted roles of antibiotics and antibiotic resistance in nature. Front Microbiol 2013; 4: 47.
        [http://dx.doi.org/10.3389/fmicb.2013.00047] [PMID: 23487476]

[7]   Antimicrobial Resistance Global Report on Surveillance. Geneva, Switzerland: World Health Organization 2014.

[8]   Andes D. Antifungal pharmacokinetics and pharmacodynamics: understanding the implications for antifungal drug resistance. Drug Resist Updat 2004; 7(3): 185-94.
        [http://dx.doi.org/10.1016/j.drup.2004.06.002] [PMID: 15296860]

[9]   Strasfeld L, Chou S. Antiviral drug resistance: mechanisms and clinical implications. Infect Dis Clin North Am 2010; 24(2): 413-37.
        [http://dx.doi.org/10.1016/j.idc.2010.01.001] [PMID: 20466277]

[10]   Margeridon-Thermet S, Shafer RW. Comparison of the Mechanisms of Drug Resistance among HIV, Hepatitis B, and Hepatitis C. Viruses 2010; 2(12): 2696-739.
        [http://dx.doi.org/10.3390/v2122696] [PMID: 21243082]

[11]   Ullman B. Multidrug resistance and P-glycoproteins in parasitic protozoa. J Bioenerg Biomembr 1995; 27(1): 77-84.
        [http://dx.doi.org/10.1007/BF02110334] [PMID: 7629055]

[12]   Greenberg RM. New approaches for understanding mechanisms of drug resistance in schistosomes. Parasitology 2013; 140(12): 1534-46.
        [http://dx.doi.org/10.1017/S0031182013000231] [PMID: 23552512]

[13]   McFadden DC, Tomavo S, Berry EA, Boothroyd JC. Characterization of cytochrome b from Toxoplasma gondii and Q(o) domain mutations as a mechanism of atovaquone-resistance. Mol Biochem Parasitol 2000; 108(1): 1-12.
        [http://dx.doi.org/10.1016/S0166-6851(00)00184-5] [PMID: 10802314]

[14]   Nagamune K, Moreno SN, Sibley LD. Artemisinin-resistant mutants of Toxoplasma gondii have altered calcium homeostasis. Antimicrob Agents Chemother 2007; 51(11): 3816-23.
        [http://dx.doi.org/10.1128/AAC.00582-07] [PMID: 17698618]

[15]   Doliwa C, Escotte-Binet S, Aubert D, *et al.* Sulfadiazine resistance in Toxoplasma gondii: no involvement of overexpression or polymorphisms in genes of therapeutic targets and ABC transporters. Parasite 2013; 20: 19.
        [http://dx.doi.org/10.1051/parasite/2013020] [PMID: 23707894]

[16]   Vanaerschot M, Dumetz F, Roy S, Ponte-Sucre A, Arevalo J, Dujardin J-C. Treatment failure in leishmaniasis: drug-resistance or another (epi-) phenotype? Expert Rev Anti Infect Ther 2014; 12(8): 937-46.
        [http://dx.doi.org/10.1586/14787210.2014.916614] [PMID: 24802998]

[17]   Mohapatra S. Drug resistance in leishmaniasis: Newer developments. Trop Parasitol 2014; 4(1): 4-9.
[http://dx.doi.org/10.4103/2229-5070.129142] [PMID: 24754020]

[18]   Yang Z, Li C, Miao M, *et al.* Multidrug-resistant genotypes of Plasmodium falciparum, Myanmar.
Emerg Infect Dis 2011; 17(3): 498-501.
[http://dx.doi.org/10.3201/eid1703.100870] [PMID: 21392443]

[19]   Bansal D, Sehgal R, Chawla Y, Malla N, Mahajan RC. Multidrug resistance in amoebiasis patients.
Indian J Med Res 2006; 124(2): 189-94.
[PMID: 17015933]

[20]   Sader HS, Castanheira M, Mendes RE, Flamm RK. Frequency and antimicrobial susceptibility of
Gram-negative bacteria isolated from patients with pneumonia hospitalized in ICUs of US medical
centres (2015-17). J Antimicrob Chemother 2018; 73(11): 3053-9.
[http://dx.doi.org/10.1093/jac/dky279] [PMID: 30060117]

CHAPTER 2

Development of Drug Resistance

Divyapriya Karthikeyan[1], Mukesh Kumar[2], Jyoti Yadav[4], Amit Alok[3], Kishore K. R. Tetala[1] and Sanjit Kumar[1,*]

[1] *Centre for Bioseparation Technology (CBST), Vellore Institute of Technology (VIT), Vellore 632014, Tamil Nadu, India*

[2] *Department of Biophysics, All India Institute of Medical Sciences, New Delhi, 110029, India*

[3] *Division of Radiation Biodosimetry, Institute of Nuclear Medicine and Allied Sciences, Timarpur, Delhi, 110054, India*

[4] *Amity Institute of Biotechnology, Amity University Rajasthan, Jaipur-303002, India*

Abstract: The phenomenon of drug resistance is a widely acknowledged problem in clinics. Drug resistance not only increases the treatment time, but also paves the way for testing the maximum limit of dose tolerance of antibiotics in the patient. There is no escaping of the fact that drug tolerance may remain a perpetual problem and bacteria will keep on evolving as a part of the natural selection process. Therefore, novel drugs targeting the novel mechanism of action could be a proposed solution for this problem. The mechanism of action includes efflux pump, alteration/modification of drug target, enzyme inactivation and prevention of drug penetration. The other thing is to avoid the unnecessary usage of antibiotics so that the bacteria living inside the body do not develop resistance. The places where antibiotics can be bought for human or animal use without a prescription, the emergence and spread of resistance are made worse. Similarly, in countries without standard treatment guidelines, antibiotics are often over-prescribed by health workers and veterinarians and over-used by the public. Therefore, this unregulated overuse of antibiotics may lead to an era where normal infection may become difficult to treat and could lead to mortality. The maintenance of hygiene is a must for everyone and it is the only way to get rid of pathogenic bacteria. So, in this chapter, we summarize recent literature on the development of drug resistance, their mechanism of actions used by microbes to develop antibiotic resistance, factors determining their development by infective agents and the spread of resistant bacteria.

Keywords: Antibiotics, Bacteria, Drug resistance.

INTRODUCTION

Drug resistance means the development of mechanisms to show less or lack of sensitivity to a particular drug or drug family. From a medical point of view, the

* **Corresponding author Sanjit Kumar:** Centre for Bioseparation Technology (CBST), Vellore Institute of Technology (VIT), Vellore 632014, Tamil Nadu, India; E-mail: sanjitkrroy@gmail.com

Sanket Kaushik and Nagendra Singh (Eds.)

increase of resistant bacterial strains is an alarming issue but at the same time, it validates the theory of adaptation in evolution. The first actual antibiotic was first discovered by Sir Alexander Fleming [1], and since then, it has been used throughout the world in medicine and plays an essential role in fighting microorganisms [2]. However, excessive use of antibiotics generated multi-resistant bacteria which pose, in recent years, a serious threat to human life [3]. A newer set of antibiotics is required to treat infections that were treated easily in the past. Bacteria surviving the hospital setup are normally drug-resistant and often require strong antibiotics with prolonged administration. Antibiotic resistance is emerging as one of the global problems to human and animal health. One year of exposure to antibacterial agents also developed resistance in many bacterial species. This is due to the constant evolution of microbes to overcome the antimicrobial compounds produced by other microorganisms and synthetic compounds [4]. The evolutionary history of pathogens reveals that antibiotics have played a pivotal role in their evolution [5]. Several important factors can accelerate the evolution of drug-resistant microbes. These include the sub-therapeutic dosing, misuse and overuse of antimicrobials, and patient noncompliance with the recommended course of treatment. This resistance develops over the due course of time due to survival mechanisms adopted by pathogen against a drug or, to a lesser extent, change in the receptor activity of a host [6, 7]. Extended usage of antibiotics has resulted in the emergence of antibiotic-resistant bacteria, which are often difficult to eradicate requiring either a higher dose or a new class of antibiotics [8].

There are several strategies used by microbes to develop antibiotic resistance which falls into the four categories such as efflux pump, alteration/modification of drug target, enzyme inactivation and prevention of drug penetration (Table 1). Although intrinsic resistance utilises efflux pump, enzyme inactivation and limited uptake of drugs and acquired resistance utilises may be drug target modification, efflux pump and enzymatic inactivation [9].

Table 1. Mechanism of drug resistance.

S.No.	Mechanism of Drug Resistance	Drug Resistant Agents
1	Efflux pump	Fluoroquinolones, aminoglycosides, tetracycline, β-lactams, macrolides
2	Alteration/modification of drug target	Fluoroquinolones, rifamycins, vancomycin, β lactams, β-lactams, aminoglycosides
3	Enzyme inactivation	β-lactams, macrolides, β-lactams, macrolides, rifamycins
4	Prevention of drug penetration	β-lactams, tetracycline, fluoroquinolones

Antibiotic resistant bacteria can modify their active site where antibiotics act, evolving a novel survival strategy [10, 11]. Researchers have also found several shreds of evidence where these microbes have an ability to inhibit the accumulation of antibiotics, thereby decreasing their effective concentration inside the bacterial cell. Bacteria produce efflux pumps to transport various antibiotic molecules. The efflux pump also flushes out antibiotics and prevent the accumulation of drug, thus, rendering bacterial resistance [12, 13]. Frequent mutations in the bacterial DNA can make the bacteria produce more pump molecules, increasing resistance. Bacteria also can change their membrane permeability. Membranes have pores that allow the transportation of molecules; thus, decreasing the permeability would mean lesser uptake of antibiotics [14, 15].

Bacteria seem to be an advanced version of this theory as some of them have developed an ability to produce enzymes that degrade antibiotics [11, 16]. Penicillin is known as the first discovered antibiotic and certain bacteria produce beta-lactamase enzymes, which degrade the beta-lactam ring of penicillin to inactivate it [17]. Some bacteria produce enzymes that are capable of adding a different chemical group to the antibiotic molecule, preventing binding between the antibiotic and its cell target. For example, *Mycobacterium tuberculosis* produces a protein that mimics the structure of DNA and this protein binds to fluoroquinolone antibiotics, thus preventing them from binding to the bacterial DNA. This property makes *M. tuberculosis* resistant to fluoroquinolones, sulphonamides, trimethoprim and DNA gyrase [18, 19].

Microbial resistance can occur in another manner when an antimicrobial drug functions as an antimetabolite by targeting a specific enzyme to inhibit its activity [20, 21]. First, bacteria may overproduce the enzymes, which are the drug targets and these target carry out enzymatic reactions. Secondly, the cell wall of bacteria develop a bypass mechanism which is not susceptible to binding of the antibiotics. Both of these strategies have been found as mechanisms of sulfonamide resistance [22, 23].

Many antibiotics act on a bacterial target (usually a protein), inactivating its activity. Some bacteria produce DNA mutations that modify the target so that these drugs may not bind to it [24]. Some bacteria add different chemical groups to the target, thus, shielding themselves from antibiotics, while some other bacteria express alternative proteins which can be used to inhibit the action of antibiotics. Hence, *Staphylococcus aureus* can produce a new penicillin-binding protein by acquiring the resistance gene *mecA* [25].

The targets of β-lactam antibiotics are proteins required for bacterial cell wall synthesis. This type of resistance is the basis of MRSA (methicillin-resistant

Staphylococcus aureus). Some bacteria have developed the ability to synthesize a new cell wall altogether for antibiotics [26]. Vancomycin-resistant bacteria have the capability to make up a different cell wall compared to susceptible bacteria. The mechanism of vancomycin-resistant among bacteria involving structural changes in peptidoglycan subunits of bacterial cell wall, prevent vancomycin from binding [22].

Pathogenic bacteria can acquire antibiotic resistance genes via vertical and horizontal gene transmission. Microbial species transfer their resistant gene to progeny and also can transfer genes between species, known as horizontal gene transfer [27 - 29]. Vertical gene transmission is an evolutionary process which occurs due to errors or mutation in the genome during replication. Horizontal gene transmission is one of the most significant dominating factors determining antimicrobial resistance. The gene responsible for antimicrobial resistance is transported through mobile genetic elements in the process of transformation, transduction, or conjugation [27]. In conjugation, two bacteria connected through structures in the cell wall and transfer DNA from one species to other. In the transduction process viruses, also known as bacteriophage take up the DNA and transfer from one bacterium to another and in transformation process, bacteria share genes by horizontal gene transfer in which bacteria can take up genetic material directly from the environment around the cell [27].

Superinfections, also known as secondary infections, due to the overuse of antibiotics in the hospital environment, have been responsible for the death of more than 5 hundred thousand individuals every year. Biofilm associated infections can also contribute to life threatening diseases such as endocarditis, rhinosinusitis and periodontitis, *etc*. Mostly biofilm formation can be observed on medical devices like urinary-catheters and medical implants [30]. Thus, preventive measures such as immunization, hygiene, intake of freshly prepared and well-cooked foods, and consulting doctors at the early stage by all individuals are the key elements to decreasing or reversing the worsening situation of antibiotic resistance [31].

In spite of creating much awareness among the public, the problem of antimicrobial resistance is alarmingly high, leading to the evolution of multi-resistant bacteria or "superbugs". To overcome this, the Longitude Prize has come up with the idea of launching a gaming app named *Superbugs*, especially for high school students. The aim of this mobile game (made with a combination of both science and fiction) is to make the individual understand how to survive and use the existing and new antimicrobials wisely [32]. Some of the solutions to this growing antimicrobial resistance are approaching new targets, drug repurposing, considering conventional drugs, combination therapy, phage therapy [33], scaling up antibiotic stewardship, reducing antibiotic use in agriculture and livestock, and using multidisciplinary approaches.

CONCLUSION

The development of antibiotic resistance is a major public health concern worldwide. In this chapter, mechanisms of development of drug resistance in bacteria have been studied. There are several mechanisms that have been discussed and are used by the microbes to develop antibiotic resistance such as alteration/modification of drug target, enzyme inactivation, efflux pump and prevention of drug penetration. The novel drugs presenting different mechanisms of action are being developed with the aim of bypassing the drug resistance phenomenon. The resistant bacteria can be transfer genetic material which are responsible for resistant not only to their same species to other bacterial species inhabiting the same environment. Transfer of antibiotic resistance can occurred by Conjugation, Transduction and Transformation. Antibiotic resistance is accelerated by the misuse and overuse of antibiotics. Biofilm formation, poor infection prevention and control can contribute to spreading infection caused by bacteria that possess resistance. Hence, it adds to the emergence of resistance, worsening the problem. There is an urgent need for action to be taken by each level of society to contain infections by resistant bacteria.

CONSENT FOR PUBLICATION

Not applicable.

CONFLICT OF INTEREST

The authors declare no conflict of interest, financial or otherwise.

ACKNOWLEDGEMENTS

S. K and Kishore acknowledge the financial assistance from the Indian Council of Medical Research (ICMR). DK thanks to ICMR for the senior research fellowship (SRF). MK thanks to ICMR for RA ship.

REFERENCES

[1]   Bennett JW, Chung K-T. Alexander Fleming and the discovery of penicillin. Elsevier 2001; pp. 163-84.
        [http://dx.doi.org/10.1016/S0065-2164(01)49013-7]

[2]   Fleming A. The discovery of penicillin. Br Med Bull 1944; 2(1): 4-5.
        [http://dx.doi.org/10.1093/oxfordjournals.bmb.a071032]

[3]   https://www.cdc.gov/drugresistance/biggest-threats.html

[4]   https://courses.lumenlearning.com/microbiology/chapter/drug-resistance/

[5]   Oz T, Guvenek A, Yildiz S, *et al.* Strength of selection pressure is an important parameter contributing to the complexity of antibiotic resistance evolution. Mol Biol Evol 2014; 31(9): 2387-401.
[http://dx.doi.org/10.1093/molbev/msu191] [PMID: 24962091]

[6]   Fish DN, Ohlinger MJ. Antimicrobial resistance: factors and outcomes. Crit Care Clin 2006; 22(2): 291-311.
[http://dx.doi.org/10.1016/j.ccc.2006.02.006] [PMID: 16678001]

[7]   Fletcher S. Understanding the contribution of environmental factors in the spread of antimicrobial resistance. Environ Health Prev Med 2015; 20(4): 243-52.
[http://dx.doi.org/10.1007/s12199-015-0468-0] [PMID: 25921603]

[8]   Meropol SB, Chan KA, Chen Z, *et al.* Adverse events associated with prolonged antibiotic use. Pharmacoepidemiol Drug Saf 2008; 17(5): 523-32.
[http://dx.doi.org/10.1002/pds.1547] [PMID: 18215001]

[9]   Reygaert WC. An overview of the antimicrobial resistance mechanisms of bacteria. AIMS microbiology. 2018;4(3):482.10. Lambert PA. Bacterial resistance to antibiotics: modified target sites. Adv Drug Deliv Rev 2005; 57(10): 1471-85.
[PMID: 15964098]

[10]   Lambert PA. Bacterial resistance to antibiotics: modified target sites. Adv Drug Deliv Rev 2005; 57(10): 1471-85.
[http://dx.doi.org/10.1016/j.addr.2005.04.002] [PMID: 15950313]

[11]   Wright GD. Bacterial resistance to antibiotics: enzymatic degradation and modification. Adv Drug Deliv Rev 2005; 57(10): 1451-70.
[http://dx.doi.org/10.1016/j.addr.2005.04.002] [PMID: 15950313]

[12]   Nikaido H, Pagès JM. Broad-specificity efflux pumps and their role in multidrug resistance of Gram-negative bacteria. FEMS Microbiol Rev 2012; 36(2): 340-63.
[http://dx.doi.org/10.1111/j.1574-6976.2011.00290.x] [PMID: 21707670]

[13]   Masi M, Réfregiers M, Pos KM, Pagès JM. Mechanisms of envelope permeability and antibiotic influx and efflux in Gram-negative bacteria. Nat Microbiol 2017; 2(3): 17001.
[http://dx.doi.org/10.1038/nmicrobiol.2017.1] [PMID: 28224989]

[14]   Ghai I, Ghai S. Understanding antibiotic resistance *via* outer membrane permeability. Infect Drug Resist 2018; 11: 523-30.
[http://dx.doi.org/10.2147/IDR.S156995] [PMID: 29695921]

[15]   Chevalier J, Pagès JM, Eyraud A, Malléa M. Membrane permeability modifications are involved in antibiotic resistance in Klebsiella pneumoniae. Biochem Biophys Res Commun 2000; 274(2): 496-9.
[http://dx.doi.org/10.1006/bbrc.2000.3159] [PMID: 10913366]

[16]   Nicoloff H, Andersson DI. Indirect resistance to several classes of antibiotics in cocultures with resistant bacteria expressing antibiotic-modifying or -degrading enzymes. J Antimicrob Chemother 2016; 71(1): 100-10.
[http://dx.doi.org/10.1093/jac/dkv312] [PMID: 26467993]

[17]   Knowles JR. Penicillin resistance: the chemistry of. beta.-lactamase inhibition. Acc Chem Res 1985; 18(4): 97-104.
[http://dx.doi.org/10.1021/ar00112a001]

[18]   Hegde SS, Vetting MW, Roderick SL, *et al.* A fluoroquinolone resistance protein from *Mycobacterium tuberculosis* that mimics DNA. Science 2005; 308(5727): 1480-3.
[http://dx.doi.org/10.1126/science.1110699] [PMID: 15933203]

[19]   Pais J, Policarpo M, Pires D, Testa B, Anesa E, Constantino L. Fluoroquinolone derivatives in the treatment of mycobacterium tuberculosis infection 2021.

[20]   Silverman R. The organic chemistry of drug design and drug action. Eur J Med Chem 1992; 27(5):

561.
[http://dx.doi.org/10.1016/0223-5234(92)90192-4]

[21]   van der Westhuyzen R, Hammons JC, Meier JL, *et al.* The antibiotic CJ-15,801 is an antimetabolite that hijacks and then inhibits CoA biosynthesis. Chem Biol 2012; 19(5): 559-71.
[http://dx.doi.org/10.1016/j.chembiol.2012.03.013] [PMID: 22633408]

[22]   McGuinness WA, Malachowa N, DeLeo FR. Vancomycin Resistance in *Staphylococcus aureus.* Yale J Biol Med 2017; 90(2): 269-81.
[PMID: 28656013]

[23]   Howden BP, Davies JK, Johnson PDR, Stinear TP, Grayson ML. Reduced vancomycin susceptibility in *Staphylococcus aureus*, including vancomycin-intermediate and heterogeneous vancomycin-intermediate strains: resistance mechanisms, laboratory detection, and clinical implications. Clin Microbiol Rev 2010; 23(1): 99-139.
[http://dx.doi.org/10.1128/CMR.00042-09] [PMID: 20065327]

[24]   Guérillot R, Li L, Baines S, *et al.* Comprehensive antibiotic-linked mutation assessment by resistance mutation sequencing (RM-seq). Genome Med 2018; 10(1): 63.
[http://dx.doi.org/10.1186/s13073-018-0572-z] [PMID: 30165908]

[25]   Wielders CLC, Fluit AC, Brisse S, Verhoef J, Schmitz FJ. mecA gene is widely disseminated in *Staphylococcus aureus* population. J Clin Microbiol 2002; 40(11): 3970-5.
[http://dx.doi.org/10.1128/JCM.40.11.3970-3975.2002] [PMID: 12409360]

[26]   Tan CM, Therien AG, Lu J, *et al.* Restoring methicillin-resistant *Staphylococcus aureus* susceptibility to β-lactam antibiotics. Sci Transl Med 2012; 4(126): 126ra35.
[http://dx.doi.org/10.1126/scitranslmed.3003592] [PMID: 22440737]

[27]   Kay E, Vogel TM, Bertolla F, Nalin R, Simonet P. In situ transfer of antibiotic resistance genes from transgenic (transplastomic) tobacco plants to bacteria. Appl Environ Microbiol 2002; 68(7): 3345-51.
[http://dx.doi.org/10.1128/AEM.68.7.3345-3351.2002] [PMID: 12089013]

[28]   Nielsen KM. Barriers to horizontal gene transfer by natural transformation in soil bacteria. APMIS Acta Pathol Microbiol Immunol Scand, Suppl 1998; 84(S84): 77-84.
[http://dx.doi.org/10.1111/j.1600-0463.1998.tb05653.x] [PMID: 9850687]

[29]   Gyles C, Boerlin P. Horizontally transferred genetic elements and their role in pathogenesis of bacterial disease. Vet Pathol 2014; 51(2): 328-40.
[http://dx.doi.org/10.1177/0300985813511131] [PMID: 24318976]

[30]   Kamaruzzaman NF, Peng TL, Hamdan RH. Biofilms-Associated Infections Continuous Challenges in Human and Animal Health 2021.

[31]   Alpert PT. Superbugs: antibiotic resistance is becoming a major public health concern. Home Health Care Manage Pract 2017; 29(2): 130-3.
[http://dx.doi.org/10.1177/1084822316659285]

[32]   https://www.nesta.org.uk/blog/our-new-game-how-long-can-you-survive-against-the-superbugs/

[33]   Viertel TM, Ritter K, Horz H-P. Viruses *versus* bacteria-novel approaches to phage therapy as a tool against multidrug-resistant pathogens. J Antimicrob Chemother 2014; 69(9): 2326-36.
[http://dx.doi.org/10.1093/jac/dku173] [PMID: 24872344]

CHAPTER 3

Current Challenges in Treating MDR

Vaishali Gurjar[1], Ayushi Khurana[1], Gunjan Shaily[1], Sanket Kaushik[2] and **Nagendra Singh[1,*]**

[1] *School of Biotechnology, Gautam Buddha University, Greater Noida, India*

[2] *Amity Institute of Biotechnology, Amity University Rajasthan, Jaipur- 303002, India*

Abstract: Multiple-Drug Resistance (MDR) is a mechanism that renders the ineffectiveness of one or more than one antimicrobial agents shown by disease causing microorganisms. MDR has become one of the major public health challenges as initially, the MDR species were restricted only to hospitals, but now they are found everywhere. Due to the slow advancements in the discovery of new or different antibiotics against the MDR organisms, the medical society is facing great challenges in the treatment of infections caused by resistant microorganisms. This chapter outlines the challenges involved in drug discovery, and treatment to fight and prevent MDR infections.

Keywords: Antibiotics, Drugs, MDR, Microorganisms, Pathogens, Proteins.

INTRODUCTION

MDR infectious microorganisms are the most threatening species to the public health as the infections caused by these organisms cannot be treated by first line antibiotics, thus resulting in more expensive and long-lasting treatments, *e.g.*, MDR-tuberculosis (TB). MDR is antimicrobial resistance expressed by a microbial species to at least one drug out of three or more antimicrobial categories [1]. Along with MDR bacteria, MDR viruses and parasites are also among the most threatening challenges to public health. Extensive drug resistance (XDR) is a new term given to microbes that are resistant to all antimicrobial agents except two or less antimicrobial categories with different chemical structures [2 - 4].

Thus, it results in a prolonged infection time and, also, adds an increased risk of infection spread. More expensive treatment options fallout with the emergence of

---

[*] **Corresponding author Nagendra Singh:** School of Biotechnology, Gautam Buddha University, Greater Noida-201308, India; E-mail: nagendratomar@gmail.com

Sanket Kaushik and Nagendra Singh (Eds.)

MDR against commercially available drugs. The evolution of global trades and tourism has increased the risk of MDR spread all over world. It is important to cutdown the use of antimicrobial agents to the lowest possible levels to reduce the risk of resistant microbes. The development of novel categories of antimicrobial agents is also desired to tackle MDR pathogens. The Infectious Diseases Society of America (IDSA) has recognized antimicrobial resistance as "one of the greatest threats to human health worldwide." MDR has a crucial impact on the lives of immunocompromised patients and has been associated with increased mortality rates. A rise in MDR has challenged all the aspects of drug designing [5, 6].

The drugs which are designed to treat a disease are target specific, any mutation in these target sites reduces the effectiveness of the particular drug, further causing antibiotic resistance. Second, the development of MDR is related to the intake of broad-spectrum antibiotics for empirical as well as definitive therapy. There are two categories of drug resistance:

Natural/Intrinsic Resistance

Few microbes show resistance towards certain drugs as they lack the metabolic process or the target sites affected by drugs. For example, vancomycin, due to its large size, cannot enter Gram-negative bacteria, as drugs in these bacteria enter through small size porins. Intrinsic resistance is also acquired by *Mycobacterium tuberculosis* for fluoroquinolones, tetracycline, aminoglycosides drugs due to the presence of efflux pumps [7].

Acquired Resistance

In a few microbes, drug resistance develops due to the consistent use of antimicrobial agents (AMA) over a period of time and or non compliance with the drug regimen. Thus, the acquired resistance depends upon the particular microorganism and the drug as well. For *e.g.*, *Staphylococci,* coliforms, and *Tubercle bacilli* are notorious microbes for rapid acquisition of resistance. Resistance in microbes may be developed by mutation (vertical transfer) or horizontal gene transfer. MDR in Mtb has been reported due to mutations, expression of genes encoding new proteins, or drug inactivating enzymes under the selection pressure of antibiotics [8].

MECHANISMS OF MDR DEVELOPMENT

Many microorganisms survive by developing adaptability to the antibiotic agents by altering their genetic makeup. Spontaneous mutations are introduced in the DNA of the microbes in order to nullify the effects of the antimicrobial agents.

This enables some bacteria to resist the activity of certain antibiotics to develop drug resistance. The mutated genes are also transferred to other microbes to make them resistant. MDR Organisms (MDROs) employ one or more mechanisms to become resistant to antibiotics.

Alteration of the Target Protein by Mutation

Mutation of a gene affected by a drug, rendering the drug ineffective, is a common way of developing resistance. The drug target site is altered as a result of spontaneous mutation of the bacterial gene on the chromosome, which gets selected in the presence of the antibiotic drug. Rifamycins and quinilones have been shown to be ineffective by mutations in the RNA polymerase and DNA gyrase genes, respectively. The resistance may also get acquired by the transfer of altered genes from one microorganism to another by transformation, conjugation or transduction, such as the acquisition of *mecA* genes responsible for methicillin resistance in *Staphylococcus aureus*.

Another example of drug resistance by the mutational changes is resistance to oxazolidinones (linezolid and tedizolid). These drugs are bacteriostatic antibiotics having a broad Gram-positive activity by binding to the A site of bacterial ribosomes and inhibiting the translation process. The mechanisms of linezolid resistance include mutations in genes encoding the domain V of the 23S rRNA and/or the ribosomal proteins L3 and L4 (rplC and rplD, respectively), and methylation of A2503 in the 23S rRNA mediated by the Cfr enzyme as modification in ribosome modulates its susceptibility to antibiotics [9].

Modifications of the Drug

One of the best bacterial strategies to develop resistance is by producing enzymes that act upon the drug and inactivate it either by its chemical modifications or by its complete destruction, rendering the drug unable to interact with target molecules.

Synthesis of enzymes responsible for chemical alteration of the drug is a well understood mechanism of acquiring resistance in both Gram-negative and Gram-positive bacteria. The most frequent biochemical alteration reactions catalysed by such enzymes are acetylation (*e.g.*, aminoglycosides, chloramphenicol, streptogramins), phosphorylation (*e.g.*, aminoglycosides, chloramphenicol), and adenylation (*e.g.*, aminoglycosides, lincosamides). The resultant reaction of target modification is hindrance in the drug binding, leading to higher bacterial minimal inhibitory concentrations (MICs) of the drugs. One of the best studied examples of this category is the presence of aminoglycoside modifying enzymes (AMEs) which catalyse covalent modification of hydroxyl or amino group of aminoglycoside antibiotics. The genes responsible for AMEs are found as part of chromosomes in several bacteria, such as some aminoglycoside acetyltransferases in *Providencia stuartii, E. faecium* and *S. marcescens*. Another example of the development of resistance by enzyme alteration is the modification of chloramphenicol. Chloramphenicol inhibits translation process by binding to the peptidyl transfer center of 50S ribosome. Chloramphenicol acetyl transferases (CATs) chemically modify the drug by acetylation. The genes encoding CATs have been found in plasmids, transposons and also as part of chromosomes in certain bacterial species [10].

Another mechanism of MDR includes the destruction of the drug molecule. The β-lactam antibiotics resistance is mainly developed by the expression of β-lactamase enzymes. These enzymes were first described in 1940s. β-lactamase hydrolyses the amide linkage in the β-lactam ring, rendering the antibiotic ineffective. Penicillinase gene responsible for resistance was found in the accessory genome of penicillin-resistant *S. aereus* bacteria. To overcome such resistance, new β-lactam drugs with a wider spectrum of activity with minimal susceptibility to penicillinase were synthesized. However, enzymes capable of degrading newer antibiotics were also found in bacteria. So far over 1,000 forms of β-lactamase genes have been found, which are expected to increase further as part of normal bacterial evolution to adapt the antimicrobial resistance.

Decreased Antibiotic Penetration and Efflux

Most clinically used antibiotics have their targets located inside the cytosol or on the inner side of the cell membrane. Therefore, an antibiotic must diffuse inside in order to exert its effects. Several bacteria have developed mechanisms to prevent antibiotic migration from outside to the periplasmic space or to the cytosol, limiting the influx of drugs. Some bacteria changed the permeability of the outer membrane, limiting the influx of polar drugs such as β-lactams, tetracyclines and some of the fluoroquinolones, which relies on membrane transporters such as aquaporins for their diffusion inside the bacterial cell. Gram-negative microorganisms developed resistance to vancomycin, a glycopeptide drug, by altering the outer cell membrane permeability. Similarly, the resistance developed by *Pseudomonas* spp. and *Acinetobacter baumanii* to β-lactams is also attributed to the reduced expression of porins in their cell membrane. The changes in porins could be achieved by various processes, such as a shift in the type of porins expressed, a change in the level of porin expression, and impairment of the porin functions [11, 12]. An example of the development of porin based resistance is the aberrant synthesis by the *OprD* gene in *P. aeruginosa*, OprD is used for the transportation of basic amino acids and antibiotics (imipenem) to the cell. *K.*

pneumonae developed resistance to β-lactams by shifting the porin expression from OmpK35 to OmpK3 (having a narrower pore size), leading to 4-8-fold decrease in the sensitivity for a wide range of β-lactam antibiotics [13]. *Neisseria gonorrhoeae* and *A. baumanii* were also found to develop resistance using a similar mechanism.

Production of the efflux pumps capable of transporting antibiotics back to extracellular milieu is another mechanism observed in many bacteria to develop antibiotic resistance. Such efflux pumps for tetracyclines were first reported in *E. coli* in early 1980s. Such mechanism affected a wide range of antibiotics such as protein synthesis inhibitors, fluoroquinolones, β-lactams, carbapenems, polymyxins, *etc.* There are 5 categories of efflux pumps reported to date, a) the major facilitator superfamily (MFS), b) the small multidrug resistance family (SMR), c) the resistance-nodulation-cell-division family (RND), d) the ATP-binding cassette family (ABC), and e) the multidrug and toxic compound extrusion family (MATE). The differ in their structures, energy sources and substrate specificities [14, 15].

Gene Acquisition from other Species for Less Susceptible Target Proteins

It is generally seen in microbes capable of natural transformation. *e.g.*, Sequencing of genes which code for the target of penicillin, penicillin binding proteins (PBPs) and DD-transpeptidase showed that penicillin resistance in *Streptococcus pneumoniae* was due to mosaic proteins production, which are originally a part of other organisms [16].

Target Bypassing

Bacteria generally avoid the action of antibiotics by interfering with their target site. This is achieved by either target protection or target site modification. In target protection, bacteria overproduce target molecules, which results in a sufficient amount of antibiotic-free target molecules to carry out the proper enzymatic reaction. In target modification, structural changes of the target molecules take place, preventing antibiotic binding. Bacteria are also capable of producing new target molecules to accomplish similar cellular functions as the original target molecules; the newer ones are not sensitive to antibiotics. Methicillin-resistant *S. aureus* acquires exogenous PBP, while vancomycin-resistant enterococci acquire resistance through modifications in their peptidoglycan structure [17]. Glycopeptides such as vancomycin and teicoplanin kill bacteria by disrupting the synthesis of the cell wall. They bind to the terminal D-alanine-D-alanine of the pentapeptide structure of the budding peptidoglycan precursors and thus preventing PBP-mediated cross-linking, resulting in inhibition of peptidoglycan cell wall synthesis. Vancomycin resistance in enterococci involves the acquisition of a group of genes (designated as *van* gene clusters) that codes for a biochemical machinery that remodels the synthesis of peptidoglycan by a) changing the last D-Ala for either D-lactate (high-level resistance) or D-serine (low-level resistance), and b) destroying the "normal" D-Ala-D-Ala ending precursors to prevent vancomycin binding to the cell wall precursors. This single replacement of D-Ala by D-lactate is responsible for 1,000-fold reduced affinity of vancomycin. Whereas, replacement by D-Ser affects interactions of antibiotics with the precursors reducing its affinity [17].

PREVENTING MDR

Strategies for treatment and prevention of MDR are an urgent requirement. The functional and controlled programmes in developing countries, such as introduction of efficient drugs and appropriate susceptibility testing, is a major requirement. TB is still the leading cause of death in the world due to a single infectious agent and still new TB cases increase at an annual rate of 2%. Fifty years ago, chemotherapy was introduced in high income countries to treat TB; however, MDR-TB has emerged, threatening TB treatment. WHO estimates that 50 million people worldwide are infected with MDR-TB [14]. For effective fight against MDR, the availability of diagnostic and therapeutic procedures within the framework of recognized standard treatment regimens should be followed as recommended by WHO. The emergence of "pan resistant" strains belonging to *Pseudomonas aeruginosa* and *Acinetobacter baumanii*, occurred more recently, also posing serious threat to MDR management. More examples are Vancomycin-Resistant Enterococci (VRE), Methicillin-resistant *Staphylococcus aureus* (MRSA), Extended-spectrum β-lactamase (ESBLs) producing Gram-negative bacteria, Klebsiella pneumoniae carbapenemase (KPC) producing Gram-negatives and Multidrug-resistant Gram negative rods (MDR GNR), MDRGN bacteria such as Enterobacter species, *E.coli*, *Klebsiella pneumoniae*, *Acinetobacter baumannii*, *Pseudomonas aeruginosa* [18].

MDR Preventive Measures

Major efforts are necessary to deal with the further rise and spread of MDR. The following measures could be adapted as per the order of preference given.

Political Commitment

Without political commitment, functionalization of a national treatment programme is impossible in a country. Awareness programmes to avoid self-medication and the only use of prescribed drugs by health professionals should be encouraged. Law should be passed to prevent the sale of unprescribed drugs. Also, health professionals should prescribe antibiotics cautiously. Education material on MDR and its prevention should be developed and distributed to the health care professionals as well as the general public and populations at risk.

Case Finding

In low income and developing countries, the cases go unreported due to expensive diagnostic methods. New diagnostic measures should be implied.

Standardized and Supervised Drug Treatment Course

Steady supply of high-quality effective drugs must be secured.

Surveillance System

Including treatment outcome monitoring, must be implemented. Improved information networking and increased corporation among stakeholders.

Development of Novel Drugs

For effective treatment should be encouraged. Research on MDR must be promoted by the science policy makers.

STRATEGIES TO COMBAT MDR

Ineffectiveness of drugs is one of the most concerning health problems globally. Mortality caused by antibiotic-resistant bacteria reached more than 23,000 deaths a year in the United States alone [20 - 25]. Hence, several measures have been adopted to tackle MDR infections. Most of them involve co-treatment with antibiotics and are not solely administered since they complement the antibiotic effect. Some of the key strategies for treatment and prevention at clinical levels are given below.

Antimicrobial Peptides (AMPs)

These are a class of small peptides that widely exists in nature. They have a wide range of inhibitory effects against pathogens. These AMPs are being studied to develop a treatment against MDR and persistent bacteria. Many AMPs are produced naturally by microbes, while few are chemically synthesized. AMPs are part of an exceptional potential strategy for combating MDR strains. AMPs have been found to have a low tendency to select for resistance, rapid killing action, broad-spectrum activity, and extraordinary clinical efficacy against many MDR bacterial species [22]. Several fungal derived defensin-like peptides, synthesized by neutrophils, have shown antimicrobial and cytotoxic properties. These AMPs were found to exhibit strong inhibitory activities against MDR *S. aureus* and persistent infections [23].

Anti-virulence Compounds

Anti-virulence compounds inhibit virulence factors in bacteria, *i.e.*, they prevent the development of infection generally without any effect on bacterial growth. Eventually anti-virulence treatment should bring into play a weaker selection for resistance compared to traditional antibiotics as they simply disable virulence factors without killing the pathogen. An acyl-depsi-peptide antibiotic, called ADEP4, is capable of activating the ClpP protease in order to kill the persistent bacterial cells. It was observed that ADEP4, along with rifampicin, is lethal for *S. aureus* biofilms [24]. Another compound called M64 was found to inhibit pro-persistence and pro-acute MvfR-dependent signalling molecules from acting against MDR strains of *P. aeruginosa* [25]. Compounds capable of reducing the formation of antibiotic tolerant persister cells have been identified. M64 block synthesis of both pro-persistence and pro-acute MvfR-dependent signaling molecules in MDR *P. aeruginosa*. BF8 ((Z)-4-bromo-5-(bromomethyle-e)-3-methylfuran-2(5H)-one) has been found to reduce persistence and revert antibiotic tolerant E. coli persister cells. BF8 is a QS inhibitor that disrupts biofilms and increases sensitivity of E. coli cells to ofloxacin [26].

Phage Therapy Alone or in Combinations with Antibiotics

To halt the spread of MDR, some alternative antibacterial therapies must emerge. Phage therapy is one of such approaches that involves the use of natural bacterial viruses (bacteriophages) which infect and cause bacterial cell lysis to treat infectious disease. Advantage of this therapy is its high target specificity towards pathogens with no adverse side-effects on host or host's microbiota. Sometimes, combined use of multiple antibiotics and phages leads to improved symptoms and a significant reduction in bacterial load, thus improving the health of the patient. Infections due to MDR strains of *A. baumannii* and *P. aeruginosa* have been treated using phage therapies [27, 28].

New Molecules

Certain new chemically-synthesized molecules such as synthetic retinoids (Vitamin A analogues), CD437 and CD1530 have been used for treating methicillin resistant *S. aeureus* (MRSA) strains, suggesting the possibility of treating MDR by disrupting the lipid bilayer. Both molecules have been found with considerable efficacy in the MRSA mouse models [29]. The carboxylic acid and the phenolic groups of the retinoids make strong, attractive interactions with the surface of the bacterial membrane bilayer, which enable retinoids to penetrate the bacterial membrane and become embedded orthogonally in the lipid molecules in the outer membrane leaflet, which perturbs the membrane integrity and changes permeability of the bacterial membrane [30].

Drug Repurposing and Repositioning

Drug discovery and development takes a long time and the success rates are generally low to enhance the fight against infection, use of non-antibiotics compounds, known as drug repurposing and repositioning is of great interest. In drug repurposing, few genes and surface proteins that are not targets of currently used antibiotics are explored. Various molecules having promising effects against MDR bacteria have been explored. Various drugs targeting nucleic acids, proteins, QS regulators, biofilm inhibitors, compounds interfering with iron metabolism are being explored to find the solution to the MDR bacteria [31 - 37].

Various types of anti-inflammatory drugs, such as acetaminophen, ibuprofen and steroids have been identified to have antimicrobial effects against red complex pathogens associated with inflammatory conditions [38]. Lieberman and Higgins identified 68 antipsychotic compounds inhibiting infection by *Listeria monocytogenes* [39]. Bepridil, a calcium channel blocker showed a neat example of repurposed drug used in the treatment of brain injury as well as to fight *L. Monocytogenes* [39]. Niclosamide (a bacteriostatic agent of salicylanilide family) was found effective against *S. aureus* resistant to methicillin, vancomycin, linezolid and daptomycin by damaging the bacterial membrane. Niclosamide was found to inhibit QS and virulence genes of *P. aeruginosa* as well [40, 41].

MDR strain of *A. baumannii* has been shown to be inhibited by three anti-ncoplastic (5-fluorouracil, 6-thioguaninc, and pifithrin-μ), an anti-rhcumatic (auranofin), an antipsychotic (fluspirilene), an anti-inflammatory and an alcohol detergent (disulfiram) compounds *in vitro* [42]. 5- fluorouracil has indicated equivalent potencies as anti cancer as well as antimicrobial agent by inhibiting thymidylate synthase enzyme. Anti-cancer drug cisplatin forms intra-strand DNA cross-links and, therefore, eradicates *E. coli* K-12, *S. aureus*, and *P. aeruginosa* persister cells through a growth-independent mechanism. Estrogen receptor modulator, Clomiphene is used to treat breast cancer. It also displays *in vitro* activity against *S. aureus*, with an MIC value of 8 mg/L [43]. Clomiphene acts by inhibiting undecaprenyl diphosphate synthase (UPPS), an enzyme involved in the synthesis of teichoic and peptidoglycan of the cell wall of *S. aureus*. Clomiphene is also known to interact with β-lactams in restoring MRSA susceptibility [44].

Lipids lowering drugs, statins act by inhibiting the human enzyme 3-hydroxy-3-methyl-glutaryl-coenzyme A reductase (HMG-CoA) leading to decreased synthesis of cholesterol and increased removal of low-density lipoprotein (LDL) circulating in the body. Statins have also shown to have antimicrobial activities against species belonging to the genera *Staphylococcus*, *Streptococcus*, *Enterococcus*, and *Moraxella* [45]. Simvastatin was able to reduce the formation and viability of mature biofilms, decreasing cell viability and extra-polysaccharide production. The antibacterial effects of statins against skin pathogens such as *S. aureus*, *E. coli*, *P. aeruginosa*, and *Serratia marcescens* are also verified using *in-vitro* studies [46].

Hand Hygiene

MDR is also known to be transferred from person-to-person by the contaminated hands of healthcare workers. Effective hand hygiene is known to be the most important measure to prevent the spread of transmissible pathogens, including MDR strains. The current disease control guidelines recommend that hands should be decontaminated by washing with antiseptic soap or with 70% ethanol. Alcohol based hand rubs are more convenient to be used [47]. WHO guidelines recommend hand hygiene to be performed before touching a patient, before clean/aseptic procedure, after body fluid exposure risk, after touching a patient and or after touching a patient's environment. Hand hygiene should always be performed before donning and after the removal of gloves. Healthcare staff must receive hand hygiene training and techniques on a regular basis [48]. Patients also should be encouraged to practice good hand hygiene in an effort to reduce environmental contamination with MDR pathogens. It is a good practice to provide a hand hygiene information leaflet to all the patients on admission.

Patient Placement and Priority for Isolation

Patients having infection with MDR microbe should be placed in isolated single rooms to avoid transmission. Dedicated staff should be given to the patients infected with MDR. It is also important to ensure that the quality of clinical care to the patient should not suffer as a result of infection control interventions such as placement in an isolation room [49]. Around each bed, there should be adequate space to minimize the spread of MDR infection to other patients. Top priority for isolation must be given to patients who have conditions to facilitate MDR transmission, *i.e.* those with uncontained secretions. 'Isolation score' may be calculated based on the type of patient and the nature of MDR infection for prioritization of the isolation [50].

Personal Protective Equipment (PPE)

PPE refers to a number of barriers that are used either alone or in combination withothers to protect healthcare workers from contact with transmissible pathogens. It includes single-use disposable gloves, aprons and long-sleeved gowns as well as facial protection for eyes, nose and mouth. PPE are removed prior to leaving the isolation room and must be discarded in appropriate heath care waste system. Hand hygiene must be performs as the final step following removal and disposable of PPE. Gloves must be worn all the time by the health care worker while contacting the MDR patient or in close proximity to the patient. Wearing gloves do not preclude the need for hand hygiene and this should always be performed after glove removal as well [51]. Disposable plastic apron or long sleeved gown and gloves should be donned before entering the room/cohort bed space of a patient infected with MDR strain. For preventing contamination, PPE should be changed between each patient in a cohort area and should be removed and discarded into an appropriate healthcare waste stream prior to leaving the patient's room [51]. After removal of PPE, hands must be decontaminated. Protection of eyes, nasal and mouth should be worn in accordance with standard precautions while dealing with patients having MDR infection.

Cleaning of the Environment and Patient Care Equipment

Environmental reservoirs such as medical equipment and surfaces play important role in the transmission of MDR strains [54]. Lack of adherence to cleaning and disinfection policies and procedures is most often a cause of environmental contamination by MDR pathogens. Interventions that help decrease the risk of MDR contamination of the environment include: Use of dedicated single-patient use medical equipment, assignment of dedicated cleaning staff to an area where patients with MDR infection are being cared for, Increased cleaning frequency and enhanced attention to frequently-touched surfaces. Monitoring for compliance with local cleaning guidelines is significant in controlling the transmission of MDR pathogens in the healthcare environment [52, 53]. The routine daily cleaning of the isolation room with detergent may be adequate, with a terminal cleaning being done on transfer/discharge of the patient as per local hospital decontamination policy. Attention should be paid to decontaminating horizontal surfaces and curtains of the area. Cleaning and disinfection of frequent touching surfaces and equipments must be done on a regular basis to avoid MDR transfer. An enhanced cleaning schedule would help at the time of any MDR pathogen outbreak in the environment.

Patient Movement and Transfer

Patients having MDR infection should have minimum movement within a facility in order to reduce the risk of cross infection. Receiving area for performing investigations and procedures should be notified in advance about MDR infection status of the patient to minimize the contact and exposure to other people. Health care staff should adopt contact precautions when caring for the patient during transfer and investigations. The clinical team should also inform the receiving staff about the MDR status of the patient while his/her transfer to another hospital or healthcare facility [53]. During surgical/invasive procedures, cleaning and disinfection of operation theatre must be carried out adequately before and after of the procedure. Appropriate signage must be placed on the door to alert staff to the use of contact precautions. The operating theatre and equipment not to be sterilised (*e.g.*, operating table) should be cleaned and disinfected between patients. The MDR patient should be cared for in a designated area within the recovery department using all contact precautions [53].

Education of Patients, Staff and Visitors

A patient should be informed about his/her MDR infection/colonization status by appropriate health documentation record by the clinical teams. Information regarding MDR pathogen and advice regarding preventing its transmission to other people also should be provided to the concerned patient. Patients are also to be encouraged about hand hygiene practices. Appropriate instructions should also be given to visitors to the patient, as well as health care workers prior to visiting the ward where a patient with MDR infection is placed.

CHALLENGES

Almost all pathogens (bacteria, virues, fungi, and parasites) show MDR enhancing their lethality rate. The development of MDR is a natural process which accelerates by the use and misuse of AMA, inappropriate handling of food, poor hygiene and poor infection control. WHO recognizes MDR as a major health threat of the 21st century [20]. The biggest challenges that are faced by the health sector are:

- To improve the current antibiotic supply.
- To develop new antibiotics for treating resistant pathogens.
- Resistant pathogens evolve their features such as impaired permeability, changes in drug target, enzymatic degradation to inactivate the antibiotic.
- Expansion of worldwide trade and tourism increases the potential of spreading MDR.
- Immunocompromised people are at a higher risk of infection.
- Treatments are becoming prolonged and expensive.

Challenges in Diagnosis

Drug resistance is essentially laboratory diagnosis since no clinical signs or symptoms are generally available for the diagnosis of MDR strains. As per WHO 2016 reports, only 57% of the pulmonary cases reports were bacteriologically confirmed [54]. The undiagnosed cases, including ones caused by drug-resistant strains, will go untreated and transmit the disease in the community. It is urgent priority to diagnose all MDR cases as early as possible in order to treat them at the earliest possible and stop community transmissions. Diagnosis of MDR strains would also require an increase in laboratory capacities worldwide in order to detect resistance to first and second line drugs in every case. However, the lack of sufficient reference laboratories in high burden countries is another big issue. Cheaper and quicker methods of detection of antimicrobial resistance (AMR) are required to be developed. In response to this challenge, high-burden countries are required to upgrade and streamline their laboratory networks. Molecular techniques should replace phenotypic methods for initial diagnosis and detection of drug resistance.

Disease Transmission

Ongoing transmission of MDR microbes generates new infections, and this infected population is the inexhaustible source of new MDR cases. In order to stop the epidemic, along with the treatment of active cases, actions are required to halt the transmission of the infection. These would require stepping up from passive case-finding to targeted active case-finding, to stop the chain of transmission, actively screening individuals at increased risk of having the infection, diagnosing them, and putting them immediately under treatment to render them non infectious. The passive case-finding approach could delay the diagnosis and the infectious period of a case, with the inevitable transmission among family members and the community by the time the case has been detected and treatment is started.

Treatment of Latent Infection

Treatment of latent infections is another major challenge in dealing with MDR. Identification of the infected individuals who could progress to active (and infectious) disease and treating their subclinical infection is crucial for interrupting the disease transmission. Providing treatment for latent infection is the chief strategy for preventing the development of active disease in patients with subclinical infections. There is no gold standard for diagnosis of latent form of tuberculosis as there is no direct measurement tool for M. *tuberculosis* infection in humans is currently available. For global elimination of MDR, pathogenesis treatment of latent infections is the key. Most of the high-burden countries have focused almost exclusively on the detection and treatment of active cases that only lead to hampering the disease elimination programs [54].

WHO'S RESPONSE TO MDR

WHO, in collaboration with Food and Agriculture Organization (FAO) of the United Nations and the World Organization for Animal Health (OIE), has developed One Health Global Action Plan to respond to antibiotic resistance [20]. As per the Global Action Plan, improvements in water sanitation and hygiene (WASH) and wastewater management in all sectors are important for the prevention of infections and reducing the spread of MDR. The objectives of the plan include 1) To improve awareness and understanding of AMR through communication, education and training, 2) To strengthen the knowledge and evidence base through surveillance and research, 3) To reduce the incidence of infection through effective sanitation, hygiene and infection prevention measures, 4) Optimize the use of antimicrobial medicines in human and animal health, 5) Develop the economic case for sustainable investment that takes account of the needs of all countries, and increase investment in new medicines, diagnostic tools, vaccines and other interventions. WHO has also urged countries to make their own action plan in view of the rapidly emerging MDR in microbes.

CONCLUSION

The ineffectiveness of more than one drug against microbes is due to MDR and the resistant pathogens are growingly becoming a challenge in the medical field of infection treatments. MDR pathogens have a crucial impact on immuno-compromised patients. Microbes produce different mechanisms to become drug resistant, which makes strategic control of MDR a necessity. Misuse of AMA and poor handling of food are among the reasons for acceleration of MDR pathogens' development. Drug repurposing is a good approach to find quicker solution to MDR s as the evaluation of drug will quickly jump to Phase II clinical trials saving time and efforts. Studies with extended clinical indications are required for the urgent need of novel methods to treat MDR pathogens. Major challenges may be confronted by essential steps such as providing sufficient funding for research and development activities, enhancing laboratory capacities, adherence to treatment and developing affordable drugs.

National disease programs in low-income countries majorly rely on international donors for their financing. The government expenditures on health care systems are less than the WHO benchmark in most the nations and most of the budgets are consumed by MDR strains in high burden countries. The extensive transmission of MDR strains is in part due to the diagnostic delays, stressing the quick need of rapid MDR detection, contact tracing and effective treatment of MDR cases. Governance and policymakers must have MDR prevention and control measures as their priority.

Especially in the high-burden states, the diagnostic laboratory capacity is urgently required to be enhanced in order to reach early stage screening of a larger number of MDR cases. The lack of adherence to treatment which leads to irregular drug intake and selection of resistant mutations, is one of the major hindrances in controlling MDR cases. Cheap and affordable drugs should be made available for high-burden and developing countries. Bedaquiline and delamanid are two drugs developed for TB in the last many years, which are also very expensive. As WHO is estimating 480,000 new cases of MDR-TB every year, it will be very difficult to manage with the unavailability of cheap and affordable drugs.

Although control of MDR has been reported using various interventions, including hand hygiene initiatives, improved education programmes, enhanced environmental cleaning, improved intra- and inter-hospital communications regarding the identification of MDR patients, there is no specific intervention or combination yet been known which could be adopted by all healthcare facilities to prevent the spread of MDR strains. More research is needed in the area of preventing and controlling MDR in the future.

CONSENT FOR PUBLICATION

Not applicable.

CONFLICT OF INTEREST

The authors declare no conflict of interest, financial or otherwise.

ACKNOWLEDGEMENTS

Declared none.

LIST OF ABBREVIATIONS

AMA	Antimicrobial agents
MDR	Multi drug resistance
TB	Tuberculosis
XDR	Extensive drug resistance
IDSA	Infectious Diseases Society of America
MDRO	MDR Organism
VRE	Vancomycin-Resistant Enterococci
MRSA	Methicillin-resistant *Staphylococcus aureus*
ESBL	Extended-spectrum β-lactamase
KPC	*Klebsiella pneumoniae* carbapenemase
AMP	Antimicrobial peptides
QS	Quoram sensor
UPPS	Undecaprenyl diphosphate synthase
LDL	Low-density lipoprotein
PPE	Personal protection equipments
AMR	Antimicrobial resistance
FAO	Food and Agriculture Organization
WASH	Water sanitation and hygiene
PBP	Penicillin binding proteins

REFERENCES

[1] Magiorakos AP, Srinivasan A, Carey RB, *et al.* Multidrug-resistant, extensively drug-resistant and pandrug-resistant bacteria: an international expert proposal for interim standard definitions for acquired resistance. Clin Microbiol Infect 2012; 18(3): 268-81.
[http://dx.doi.org/10.1111/j.1469-0691.2011.03570.x] [PMID: 21793988]

[2] Medina E, Pieper DH. Tackling threats and future problems of multidrug-resistant bacteria. Curr Top Microbiol Immunol 2016; 398: 3-33.
[http://dx.doi.org/10.1007/82_2016_492] [PMID: 27406189]

[3] Munita JM, Arias CA. Mechanisms of antibiotic resistance. Microbiol Spectr 2016; 4(2): 10.
[http://dx.doi.org/10.1128/microbiolspec.VMBF-0016-2015] [PMID: 27227291]

[4] Tanwar J, Das S, Fatima Z, Hameed S. Multidrug resistance: an emerging crisis. Interdiscip Perspect Infect Dis 2014; 2014: 541340.
[http://dx.doi.org/10.1155/2014/541340] [PMID: 25140175]

[5] Spellberg B, Blaser M, Guidos RJ, *et al.* Combating antimicrobial resistance: policy recommendations to save lives. Clin Infect Dis 2011; 52 (Suppl. 5): S397-428.
[http://dx.doi.org/10.1093/cid/cir153] [PMID: 21474585]

[6] Cassini A, Högberg LD, Plachouras D, *et al.* Attributable deaths and disability-adjusted life-years caused by infections with antibiotic-resistant bacteria in the EU and the European Economic Area in 2015: A population-level modelling analysis. Lancet Infect Dis 2018; 19(1): 55-6.
[http://dx.doi.org/10.1016/S1473-3099(18)30605-4] [PMID: 30409683]

[7]   McMurry L, Petrucci RE Jr, Levy SB. Active efflux of tetracycline encoded by four genetically different tetracycline resistance determinants in Escherichia coli. Proc Natl Acad Sci 1980; 77(7): 3974-7.

[8]   Culyba MJ, Mo CY, Kohli RM. Targets for combating the evolution of acquired antibiotic resistance. Biochemistry 2015; 54(23): 3573-82.
[http://dx.doi.org/10.1021/acs.biochem.5b00109] [PMID: 26016604]

[9]   Stojković V, Noda-Garcia L, Tawfik DS, Fujimori DG. Antibiotic resistance evolved *via* inactivation of a ribosomal RNA methylating enzyme. Nucleic Acids Res 2016; 44(18): 8897-907.
[http://dx.doi.org/10.1093/nar/gkw699] [PMID: 27496281]

[10]   Lambert PA. Bacterial resistance to antibiotics: modified target sites. Adv Drug Deliv Rev 2005; 57(10): 1471-85.
[http://dx.doi.org/10.1016/j.addr.2005.04.003] [PMID: 15964098]

[11]   Doménech-Sánchez A, Martínez-Martínez L, Hernández-Allés S, *et al.* Role of *Klebsiella pneumoniae* OmpK35 porin in antimicrobial resistance. Antimicrob Agents Chemother 2003; 47(10): 3332-5.
[http://dx.doi.org/10.1128/AAC.47.10.3332-3335.2003] [PMID: 14506051]

[12]   Quinn JP, Dudek EJ, DiVincenzo CA, Lucks DA, Lerner SA. Emergence of resistance to imipenem during therapy for *Pseudomonas aeruginosa* infections. J Infect Dis 1986; 154(2): 289-94.
[http://dx.doi.org/10.1093/infdis/154.2.289] [PMID: 3088133]

[13]   Hasdemir UO, Chevalier J, Nordmann P, Pagès JM. Detection and prevalence of active drug efflux mechanism in various multidrug-resistant Klebsiella pneumoniae strains from Turkey. J Clin Microbiol 2004; 42(6): 2701-6.
[http://dx.doi.org/10.1128/JCM.42.6.2701-2706.2004] [PMID: 15184455]

[14]   Pagès JM, James CE, Winterhalter M. The porin and the permeating antibiotic: a selective diffusion barrier in Gram-negative bacteria. Nat Rev Microbiol 2008; 6(12): 893-903.
[http://dx.doi.org/10.1038/nrmicro1994] [PMID: 18997824]

[15]   Piddock LJ. Clinically relevant chromosomally encoded multidrug resistance efflux pumps in bacteria. Clin Microbiol Rev 2006; 19(2): 382-402.
[http://dx.doi.org/10.1128/CMR.19.2.382-402.2006] [PMID: 16614254]

[16]   Spratt BG. Resistance to antibiotics mediated by target alterations. Science 1994; 264(5157): 388-93.
[http://dx.doi.org/10.1126/science.8153626] [PMID: 8153626]

[17]   Miller WR, Munita JM, Arias CA. Mechanisms of antibiotic resistance in enterococci. Expert Rev Anti Infect Ther 2014; 12(10): 1221-36.
[http://dx.doi.org/10.1586/14787210.2014.956092] [PMID: 25199988]

[18]   Boucher HW, Talbot GH, Bradley JS, *et al.* Bad bugs, no drugs: no ESKAPE! An update from the Infectious Diseases Society of America. Clin Infect Dis 2009; 48(1): 1-12.
[http://dx.doi.org/10.1086/595011] [PMID: 19035777]

[19]   Menzies NA, Cohen T, Lin HH, Murray M, Salomon JA. Population health impact and cost-effectiveness of tuberculosis diagnosis with Xpert MTB/RIF: a dynamic simulation and economic evaluation. PLoS Med 2012; 9(11): e1001347.
[http://dx.doi.org/10.1371/journal.pmed.1001347] [PMID: 23185139]

[20]   World Health Organization. Global action plan on antimicrobial resistance 2015. Avilable from https://www.who.int/publications/i/item/9789241509763

[21]   Singh V. "Antimicrobial resistance," in Microbial Pathogens and Strategies for Combating Them: Science, Technology and Education. Formatex Research Center 2013; 1: 291-6.

[22]   Mwangi J, Hao X, Lai R, Zhang ZY. Antimicrobial peptides: new hope in the war against multidrug resistance. Zool Res 2019; 40(6): 488-505.
[http://dx.doi.org/10.24272/j.issn.2095-8137.2019.062] [PMID: 31592585]

[23] Yang N, Teng D, Mao R, *et al.* A recombinant fungal defensin-like peptide-P2 combats multidrug-resistant *Staphylococcus aureus* and biofilms. Appl Microbiol Biotechnol 2019; 103(13): 5193-213.
[http://dx.doi.org/10.1007/s00253-019-09785-0] [PMID: 31025073]

[24] Conlon BP, Nakayasu ES, Fleck LE, *et al.* Activated ClpP kills persisters and eradicates a chronic biofilm infection. Nature 2013; 503(7476): 365-70.
[http://dx.doi.org/10.1038/nature12790] [PMID: 24226776]

[25] Starkey M, Lepine F, Maura D, *et al.* Identification of anti-virulence compounds that disrupt quorum-sensing regulated acute and persistent pathogenicity. PLoS Pathog 2014; 10(8): e1004321.
[http://dx.doi.org/10.1371/journal.ppat.1004321] [PMID: 25144274]

[26] Pan J, Xie X, Tian W, *et al.* (Z)-4-bromo-5-(bromomethylene)-3-methylfuran-2(5H)-one sensitizes *Escherichia coli* persister cells to antibiotics. Appl Microbiol Biotechnol 2013; 97(20): 9145-54.
[http://dx.doi.org/10.1007/s00253-013-5185-2] [PMID: 24006079]

[27] Schooley RT, Biswas B, Gill JJ, *et al.* Development and use of personalized bacteriophage-based therapeutic cocktails to treat a patient with a disseminated resistant acinetobacter baumannii infection. Antimicrob Agents Chemother 2017; 61(10): e00954-17.
[http://dx.doi.org/10.1128/AAC.00954-17] [PMID: 28807909]

[28] Khawaldeh A, Morales S, Dillon B, *et al.* Bacteriophage therapy for refractory *Pseudomonas aeruginosa* urinary tract infection. J Med Microbiol 2011; 60(Pt 11): 1697-700.
[http://dx.doi.org/10.1099/jmm.0.029744-0] [PMID: 21737541]

[29] Kim W, Zhu W, Hendricks GL, *et al.* A new class of synthetic retinoid antibiotics effective against bacterial persisters. Nature 2018; 556(7699): 103-7.
[http://dx.doi.org/10.1038/nature26157] [PMID: 29590091]

[30] Pacios O, Blasco L, Bleriot I, *et al.* Strategies to combat multidrug-resistant and persistent infectious diseases. Antibiotics (Basel) 2020; 9(2): 65.
[http://dx.doi.org/10.3390/antibiotics9020065] [PMID: 32041137]

[31] Domínguez AV, Mejías MEJ, Smani Y. Drugs Repurposing for Multi-Drug Resistant Bacterial Infections. 2020.
[http://dx.doi.org/10.5772/intechopen.93635]

[32] Cruz-Muñiz MY, LópezJacome LE, Hernández-Durán M, Franco-Cendejas R. Repurposing the anticancer drug mitomycin C for the treatment of persistent Acinetobacter baumannii infections. Int J Antimicrobial Agents 2017; 49(1): 88-92.

[33] Domalaon R, Ammeter D, Brizuela M, Gorityala BK, Zhanel GG, Schweizer F. Repurposed antimicrobial combination therapy: Tobramycin-ciprofloxacin hybrid augments activity of the anticancer drug mitomycin C against multidrug-resistant Gram-negative bacteria. Front Microbiol 2019; 10: 1556.
[http://dx.doi.org/10.3389/fmicb.2019.01556] [PMID: 31354660]

[34] Kwan BW, Chowdhury N, Wood TK. Combatting bacterial infections by killing persister cells with mitomycin C. Environ Microbiol 2015; 17(11): 4406-14.
[http://dx.doi.org/10.1111/1462-2920.12873] [PMID: 25858802]

[35] Thangamani S, Younis W, Seleem MN. Repurposing celecoxib as a topical antimicrobial agent. Front Microbiol 2015; 6(7): 750.
[http://dx.doi.org/10.3389/fmicb.2015.00750] [PMID: 26284040]

[36] She P, Wang Y, Luo Z, *et al.* Meloxicam inhibits biofilm formation and enhances antimicrobial agents efficacy by *Pseudomonas aeruginosa*. MicrobiologyOpen 2018; 7(1): e00545.
[http://dx.doi.org/10.1002/mbo3.545] [PMID: 29178590]

[37] Rezzoagli C, Wilson D, Weigert M, Wyder S, Kümmerli R. Probing the evolutionary robustness of two repurposed drugs targeting iron uptake in *Pseudomonas aeruginosa*. Evol Med Public Health 2018; 2018(1): 246-59.

[http://dx.doi.org/10.1093/emph/eoy026] [PMID: 30455950]

[38]   Vijayashree Priyadharsini J. *In silico* validation of the non-antibiotic drugs acetaminophen and ibuprofen as antibacterial agents against red complex pathogens. J Periodontol 2019; 90(12): 1441-8.
[http://dx.doi.org/10.1002/JPER.18-0673] [PMID: 31257588]

[39]   Lieberman LA, Higgins DE. Inhibition of *Listeria monocytogenes* infection by neurological drugs. Int J Antimicrob Agents 2010; 35(3): 292-6.
[http://dx.doi.org/10.1016/j.ijantimicag.2009.10.011] [PMID: 20031379]

[40]   Rajamuthiah R, Fuchs BB, Conery AL, *et al.* Repurposing salicylanilide anthelmintic drugs to combat drug resistant *Staphylococcus aureus*. PLoS One 2015; 10(4): e0124595.
[http://dx.doi.org/10.1371/journal.pone.0124595] [PMID: 25897961]

[41]   Imperi F, Massai F, Ramachandran Pillai C, *et al.* New life for an old drug: the anthelmintic drug niclosamide inhibits *Pseudomonas aeruginosa* quorum sensing. Antimicrob Agents Chemother 2013; 57(2): 996-1005.
[http://dx.doi.org/10.1128/AAC.01952-12] [PMID: 23254430]

[42]   Cheng YS, Sun W, Xu M, *et al.* Repurposing Screen Identifies Unconventional Drugs With Activity Against Multidrug Resistant *Acinetobacter baumannii*. Front Cell Infect Microbiol 2019; 8: 438.
[http://dx.doi.org/10.3389/fcimb.2018.00438] [PMID: 30662875]

[43]   Chowdhury N, Wood TL, Martínez-Vázquez M, García-Contreras R, Wood TK. DNA-crosslinker cisplatin eradicates bacterial persister cells. Biotechnol Bioeng 2016; 113(9): 1984-92.
[http://dx.doi.org/10.1002/bit.25963] [PMID: 26914280]

[44]   Farha MA, Czarny TL, Myers CL, *et al.* Antagonism screen for inhibitors of bacterial cell wall biogenesis uncovers an inhibitor of undecaprenyl diphosphate synthase. Proc Natl Acad Sci USA 2015; 112(35): 11048-53.
[http://dx.doi.org/10.1073/pnas.1511751112] [PMID: 26283394]

[45]   Jerwood S, Cohen J. Unexpected antimicrobial effect of statins. J Antimicrob Chemother 2008; 61(2): 362-4.
[http://dx.doi.org/10.1093/jac/dkm496] [PMID: 18086693]

[46]   Ko HHT, Lareu RR, Dix BR, Hughes JD. *In vitro* antibacterial effects of statins against bacterial pathogens causing skin infections. Eur J Clin Microbiol Infect Dis 2018; 37(6): 1125-35.
[http://dx.doi.org/10.1007/s10096-018-3227-5] [PMID: 29569046]

[47]   Boyce JM, Pittet D. HICPAC/SHEA/APIC/IDSA Hand Hygiene Task Force. Guidelines for Hand Hygiene in Health-Care Settings. Recommendations of the Healthcare Infection Control Practices Advisory Committee and the HICPAC/SHEA/APIC/IDSA Hand Hygiene Task Force. Society for Healthcare Epidemiology of America/Association for Professionals in Infection Control/Infectious Diseases Society of America. MMWR Recomm Rep 2002; 51(RR-16): 1-45.
[PMID: 12418624]

[48]   SARI (Strategy for the Control of Antimicrobial Resistance in Ireland) Infection control subcommittee.. Guidelines for Hand Hygiene in the Irish Healthcare Setting 2005. Available from http://www.hpsc.ie/hpsc/A-Z/Gastroenteric/Handwashing/ Publications/File,1047,en.pdf

[49]   Cookson BD, Macrae MB, Barrett SP, *et al.* Guidelines for the control of glycopeptide-resistant enterococci in hospitals. J Hosp Infect 2006; 62(1): 6-21.
[http://dx.doi.org/10.1016/j.jhin.2005.02.016] [PMID: 16310890]

[50]   Auckland C, Pallett A, Smith J. Use of adult isolation facilities in a UK infectious diseases unit. J Hosp Infect 2002; 52(1): 74-5.
[http://dx.doi.org/10.1053/jhin.2002.1242] [PMID: 12372333]

[51]   From the Public Health Service US Department of Health and Human Services Centres for Disease Control and Prevention Atlanta Georgia. 2007.

[52]   CDC, Healthcare Infection Control Practices Advisory Committee. 2007. Available from

http://www.cdc.gov/ncidod/dhqp/pdf/ar/mdroguideline2006

[53] Tacconelli E, Cataldo MA, Dancer SJ, *et al.* ESCMID guidelines for the management of the infection control measures to reduce transmission of multidrug-resistant Gram-negative bacteria in hospitalized patients. Clin Microbiol Infect 2014; 20 (Suppl. 1): 1-55.
[http://dx.doi.org/10.1111/1469-0691.12427] [PMID: 24329732]

[54] Laniado-Laborín R. Clinical challenges in the era of multiple and extensively drug-resistant tuberculosis. Rev Panam Salud Publica 2017; 41: e167.
[http://dx.doi.org/10.26633/RPSP.2017.167] [PMID: 31384279]

CHAPTER 4

Methods of Detection of MDR

Monish Bisen[1], Anupam Jyoti[2] and **Juhi Saxena[2,*]**

[1] *Faculty of Applied Sciences and Biotechnology, Shoolini University of Biotechnology and Management Sciences, Bajhol, Solan, Himachal Pradesh 173229, India*

[2] *Department of Biotechnology, University Institute of Biotechnology, Chandigarh University, Mohali, Punjab, 140413, India*

Abstract: World health organization (WHO) has acknowledged the problem of multi-drug resistance (MDR) bacteria as an endemic and widespread problem globally. MDR in LMICs represents one of the biggest threats to global health and is one of the greatest current challenges in infectious disease research. High mortality/morbidity rates of MDR infections are mainly due to the lack of timely, rapid detection and treatment of the causative pathogen. Molecular mechanism conferring MDR against most common treatment options includes mutations in antibiotics' susceptible genes at one or many sites. A number of methods, including culture-based, nucleic acid-based amplification of resistance conferring genes, and immunological based assays have been developed to detect MDR. Each method has defined specificity, sensitivity and time around to detect MDR infections in clinical settings.

Keywords: Antimicrobial Resistance, Detection of MDR, Multi-drug resistance bacteria (MDR), MDR infections.

INTRODUCTION

Emergence of multi-drug resistance bacteria (MDR) is a serious threat to global health care system. These 'superbugs' are ubiquitously present, causing mortality worldwide. Pathogen showing insensitivity to at least one in three or more antimicrobial categories is termed to be MDR. The development of resistant strains is explained well by natural selection theory. Irrational use of antibiotics, poor sanitation, inapt food and hygiene practices cause sensitive bacteria to divide and mutate. Such mutated strains transfer their resistant genes over the generations (Table **1**). Infections due to MDR bacteria are of serious concern as

* **Corresponding author Juhi Saxena:** Department of Biotechnology, University Institute of Biotechnology, Chandigarh University, Mohali, Punjab, 140413, India; E-mail: jina.saxena@gmail.com

Sanket Kaushik and Nagendra Singh (Eds.)

very few treatment options are available with current antibiotic therapy. Moreover, such mutated strains are the main culprits for the spread and outbreak of antibiotic resistance. Penicillin-resistant *Streptococcus pneumoniae*, Methicillin-resistant *Staphylococcus aureus* are common Gram-positive bacteria. Vancomycin-Resistant *Enterococci*, Extended-spectrum β-lactamase *Klebsiella pneumoniae* (carbapenemase) represent Gram-negatives. Including bacteria, all other infectious agents like viruses, fungi, parasites, protozoans are capable of developing and spreading antimicrobial resistance. In primary, secondary or clinical MDR, the problems get terribly worse in the immune comprised host, subsequently leading to persistent illness and high therapeutic cost [1].

Table 1. Prevalent drug-resistant microbes.

S. No	Name of Bacterium	Drug	Genes	References
1.	*Escherichia coli*	Carbapenem and Cephalosporins	*Tem*	[3]
2.	*Enterobacter spp.*	Carbapenem	*Tem*	[4]
3.	*Klebsiella spp.*	Carbapenem, Colistin, and Cephalosporins	*tem, ctxM, vanB, shv, blaKPC1*	[5]
4.	*Acinetobacter baumannii*	Carbapenem	*Tem*	[6]
5.	*Pseudomonas aeruginosa*	Carbapenem	*Tem*	[7]
6.	*Staphylococcus aureus*	Methicillin	*vanA, mec*	[8]
7.	*Enterococcus faecium*	Vancomycin	*vanB, vanC*	[9]
8.	*Salmonella* Typhi	Fluoroquinolone	*invA,hilA*	[10]
9.	*Streptococcus pneumoniae*	Penicillin	*parC, gyrA*	[11]
10.	*Neisseria gonorrhoeae*	Cephalosporins	*gyrA*	[12]
11.	*Mycobacterium tuberculosis*	Rifampicin, isoniazid, and fluoroquinolone	*katG, rpoB*	[13]

MDR bacteria have shown a myriad of strategies to reduce the efficacy of available drugs. Genetic mutations, exchange of plasmid or chromosomal genes, reformed cell wall composition and permeability, target proteins or enzymes modifications, efflux pumps, enzymatic antimicrobial inactivation or transformation are some of them. As per the WHO's reports (2020), the mortal combat against these multi-drug resistance bacteria is a big concern and presents a multitude of challenges with very few effective and innovative antibiotics. By 2050, no treatment options will be available against these MDR bacteria. Looking at the present scenario, immediate screening of drug resistance and new alternatives for treatment hold paramount significance [2].

*According to a report on anti-tuberculosis drug resistance in the world prepared by the WHO/IUATLD Global Project on anti-tuberculosis drug-resistance surveillance, MDR-TB has reached rates of up to 14% among new patients and up to 50% in previously-treated patients in some contexts (World Health Organization, 2004).

TECHNIQUES TO DETECT MDR

A number of techniques have been devised to detect MDR bacteria. This chapter will evaluate the different methods to detect MDR pathogens (Fig. **1**).

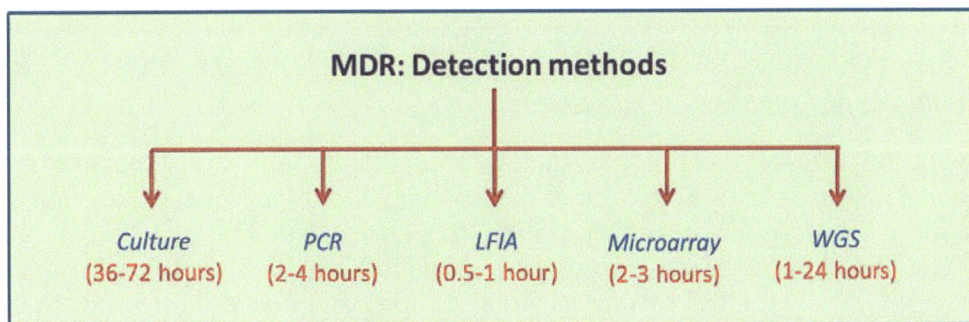

MDR: Detection methods

| Culture (36-72 hours) | PCR (2-4 hours) | LFIA (0.5-1 hour) | Microarray (2-3 hours) | WGS (1-24 hours) |

Fig. (1). Different methods to detect multi-drug resistance (MDR) along with their detection time range. PCR: Polymerase Chain Reaction; LFIA: Lateral Flow Immuno-Assay; WGS: Whole Gene Sequencing. See text for details.

Culture

Culture based methods are the gold standard for not only identification but also for the detection of MDR bacteria. Identification of bacteria is the first step in the antibacterial susceptibility test (AST). This is done by microdilution of suspected blood followed by plating to obtain a pure culture of bacteria. The bacteria are identified by Gram staining and biochemical tests as standard methods. After identification, bacteria are subjected to AST, where bacterial isolates are allowed to grow in the presence of a known concentration of antibiotics and their growth is monitored by visual detection. Nowadays, various AST cards and wells having known concentration of specific antibiotics are commercially available, which monitor the growth as well as resistivity/sensitivity pattern of bacteria against antibiotics. Despite this, culture based MDR detection method takes 3 to 5 days to get a conclusive result, and by that time, patients are administered broad-spectrum antibiotics, which further leads to the development of MDR and poor patient outcome. Hence, newer methods have been developed to improve the sensitivity and specificity as well as reduce the sample processing and MDR detection time [14].

Culture based detection method falls in the category of phenotypic methods, such as:

Liquid Culture-based Methods

Several liquid culture-based approaches for *M. tuberculosis* cultivation and drug susceptibility testing (DST) have been introduced in recent years. The majority of them are commercially accessible and rely on the fact that liquid media allows for faster development. Some are simple manual processes, while others rely on more advanced automated technologies. In low- and middle-income countries, WHO recommendations support the use of liquid culture media for M. tuberculosis cultivation and DST (World Health Organization, 2007).

Advantages of Liquid-culture Method

Among the different technologies that are available, liquid culture methods have attracted a lot of attention because of their potential to improve case detection and provide rapid drug susceptibility testing (DST) for both first- and second-line medications. Although liquid culture has benefits, it is also vital to consider its complexity, evaluate the reasons for implementing automated liquid culture, and ensure that it is an appropriate first reaction to laboratory strengthening in the local environment [21].

Solid-culture Methods

New solid culture media-based approaches for quick DST of M. tuberculosis have also recently been proposed. The majority of these alternate techniques were created as 'in-house' approaches to reduce the Turnaround time (TAT) to obtain final results [19].

Advantages of Solid-culture

Solid culture media make it easier to detect contaminants and choose the proper colony for further analysis. In addition, the morphology of colonies makes it easier to distinguish between species in mixed infections [22].

In solid media, utilising an inverted microscope or an autofluorescence detector to detect fluorescence light emitted by the organism can help with naked-eye detection of colonies in the TLA [23].

Culture-based approaches have the disadvantage of taking a long time to provide conclusive results, which can take days.

Polymerase Chain Reaction

Polymerase chain reaction (PCR) is the most reliable and powerful tool which enables the detection of MDR by amplifying and detecting antimicrobial resistance (AMR) genes. A number of bacteria express AMR genes, which confer them resistant against selective antibiotics (Table **1**). PCR-based diagnosis is the first suggested measure for asymptomatic and symptomatic patients having a heavy MDR infection burden. Consumables need proper storage conditions, but the equipment is automated and can easily be used in laboratories. Multiplex PCR, the advanced version, offers higher specificity and is used to detect many resistance marker genes in a single run time. With the advent of emerging drug resistant variants, several modifications of the PCR technique have been established to recognize exact copy numbers of MDR pathogens. Nowadays, many labs are employing real time PCR (rtPCR) followed by high resolution melt curve analysis, which is able to detect even a single mutation in the antibiotic sensitive gene. Sequence-specific probes are used to amplify target drug-resistance genes. Pre-requisites for PCR-based detection of MDR genes is the knowledge of complete sequence of MDR genes. Hence, this technique is limited to targeted bacteria. Additionally, this technique requires expensive equipment, reagents and trained man power [15].

Advantages

The ability to distinguish and quantify only living organisms is a benefit of quantitative real-time polymerase chain reaction (qPCR) and reverse transcriptase (RT-qPCR). Loop Mediated Isothermal Amplification (LAMP), the third approach, has various advantages over PCR procedures, including a moderate-temperature amplification strategy that allows for simple and cost-effective equipment. Using four primers and the strand-displacement activity of Bst DNA polymerase, great specificity is achieved in a quick and robust single-step amplification (avoiding high temperature denaturation) that allows direct detection of DNA at 60–65 1C in 15–60 minutes from nearly raw samples [20].

Disadvantages

Only the genes targeted in the assay can be identified, which is a drawback. As a result, with the discovery of novel resistance genes, multiplex PCR must be continuously enhanced and enlarged [24].

Lateral Flow Immunoassay

Lateral flow immunoassay (LFIA) relies on antibody-based detection of proteins coded by MDR genes. LFIA is a miniatured strip-based assay where a test sample in the form of liquid is added to one end of the strip and allowed to migrate by capillary action to the other end. Specific antibody against the MDR protein is conjugated with chromogen and adhered to the membrane of the strip. This method is rapid, highly cost-effective, and can detect multiple MDR proteins in a single strip. However, the pre-requisite to this method is that it requires liquid media; hence culture step is required [16].

Advantages

The lateral flow immunoassay is one of the most extensively used immunoassays in on-site detection. It offers a simple strip test that uses a nanoparticle-labeled antibody probe to detect the sample rapidly and without the need for expensive equipment or trained analysts. Aside from its high sensitivity and specificity, this approach also has the advantage of being simple to use, making it a viable option for a preliminary screening kit. The screening needed only two steps: adding bacterial solution and checking the result displayed by the device, obviating the requirement for experienced laboratory technicians and allowing for high-throughput screening [25].

Disadvantages

In remote locations, reaction reagents are prohibitively expensive. As a result, developing speedy and effective detection methods is critical [26].

DNA Microarray

DNA microarray, a hybridization-based assay, is used to detect MDR genes by pairing them to the labelled probes. In this method, single-stranded DNA of known MDR gene sequences is fixed in designated spots on glass plates. Sample containing MDR genes to be detected denatured to get single stranded form and labelled with a fluorescent marker. Furthermore, the sample is loaded on arrays having known single stranded probe and allowed to hybridize. Spots showing fluorescence is detected with a scanner and designated as a positive sample for MDR bacteria. The major advantage of this method is that in a single platform, various MDR pathogens can be detected. However, this method also requires specialized equipment which is costly, hence limiting its utility in clinics [17].

Advantages

When compared to the Xpert MTB/RIF assays, the microarray system has two benefits. First, because the Xpert MTB/RIF cartridges are disposable, the microarray assay is less expensive. Second, the microarray assay can detect both RMP and INH-related gene mutations [27].

Disadvantages

There are certain drawbacks to these DNA microarrays. Short oligonucleotide arrays printed on glass slides are more specific, but they come at a higher cost due to the need for modified oligonucleotides, and samples may need to be amplified with specific primers during labelling, which would be problematic for an array designed to detect nearly 1,000 genes [30].

Whole Genome Sequencing

Whole genome sequencing (WGS) is instrumental in detecting MDR genes of targeted and untargeted pathogens, which could not be possible by PCR and microarray. A number of techniques including Sanger, Illumina, PacBio, and Nanopore have been developed, which can detect MDR pathogens rapidly with increased sensitivity as well as specificity. The major problem which limits its widespread use in clinics is the high equipment cost, trained man power, and need for bioinformatician to analyze the data [18].

Advantages

Whole genome sequencing provides the advantage of knowing the whole DNA sequence of an organism's genome and discovering drug resistance-inducing mutations, including those associated with the novel drug, all at once, allowing for a more appropriate and accurate regimen selection [29].

Disadvantages

The most extensively utilized WGS solution is Illumina sequencing technology. The short reads, which prevent resolution of large-repeat/low-complexity areas, and the potential of incomplete base extensions (phasing and prephasing), which together increase final error rates, are downsides of this method [28].

CONCLUSIONS

MDR is a serious alarm to global public health and is rising every day. Hence, there is an urgent need to detect MDR so that appropriate antibiotics can be administered to the suspected patients for a better outcome. Keeping this in mind, a number of techniques, including PCR, microarray, LFIA, and WGS have been developed. All these techniques have advantages and limitations. Further research is required to reduce their shortcomings so that these can be routinely used in clinics.

Microorganisms have evolved and developed resistance to existing antibiotics throughout time. This has caused a significant impact on the world's health and socioeconomic conditions. They are acquiring resistance at such a rapid rate that present pharmaceutical technology and new therapeutic innovations are unable to keep up.

CONSENT FOR PUBLICATION

Not applicable.

CONFLICT OF INTEREST

The authors declare no conflict of interest, financial or otherwise.

ACKNOWLEDGEMENTS

We acknowledge Chandigarh University, Mohali for offering support and encouragement all through the work.

REFERENCES

[1]   Vivas R, Barbosa AAT, Dolabela SS, Jain S. Multidrug-resistant bacteria and alternative methods to control them: an overview. Microb Drug Resist 2019; 25(6): 890-908.
[http://dx.doi.org/10.1089/mdr.2018.0319] [PMID: 30811275]

[2]   Global Antimicrobial Resistance Surveillance System (GLASS): molecular methods for antimicrobial resistance (AMR) diagnostics to enhance the Global Antimicrobial Resistance Surveillance System. World Health Organization 2019.

[3]   Pfeifer Y, Cullik A, Witte W. Resistance to cephalosporins and carbapenems in Gram-negative bacterial pathogens. Int J Med Microbiol 2010; 300(6): 371-9.
[http://dx.doi.org/10.1016/j.ijmm.2010.04.005] [PMID: 20537585]

[4]   Bratu S, Landman D, Alam M, Tolentino E, Quale J. Detection of KPC carbapenem-hydrolyzing enzymes in Enterobacter spp. from Brooklyn, New York. Antimicrob Agents Chemother 2005; 49(2): 776-8.
[http://dx.doi.org/10.1128/AAC.49.2.776-778.2005] [PMID: 15673765]

[5]   Yigit H, Queenan AM, Anderson GJ, *et al.* Novel carbapenem-hydrolyzing β-lactamase, KPC-1, from a carbapenem-resistant strain of Klebsiella pneumoniae. Antimicrob Agents Chemother 2008; 52(2): 809.
[http://dx.doi.org/10.1128/AAC.01445-07] [PMID: 11257029]

[6]   Krizova L, Poirel L, Nordmann P, Nemec A. TEM-1 β-lactamase as a source of resistance to sulbactam in clinical strains of Acinetobacter baumannii. J Antimicrob Chemother 2013; 68(12): 2786-91.
[http://dx.doi.org/10.1093/jac/dkt275] [PMID: 23838947]

[7]   Bahrami M, Mmohammadi-Sichani M, Karbasizadeh V. Prevalence of SHV, TEM, CTX-M and OXA-48 β-Lactamase Genes in Clinical Isolates of *Pseudomonas aeruginosa* in Bandar-Abbas, Iran. Avicenna J Clin Microbiol Infect 2018; 5(4): 86-90.

[http://dx.doi.org/10.34172/ajcmi.2018.18]

[8]   Ghahremani M, Jazani NH, Sharifi Y. Emergence of vancomycin-intermediate and -resistant *Staphylococcus aureus* among methicillin-resistant *S. aureus* isolated from clinical specimens in the northwest of Iran. J Glob Antimicrob Resist 2018; 14: 4-9.
[http://dx.doi.org/10.1016/j.jgar.2018.01.017] [PMID: 29454049]

[9]   Messi P, Guerrieri E, de Niederhäusern S, Sabia C, Bondi M. Vancomycin-resistant enterococci (VRE) in meat and environmental samples. Int J Food Microbiol 2006; 107(2): 218-22.
[http://dx.doi.org/10.1016/j.ijfoodmicro.2005.08.026] [PMID: 16280183]

[10]   Wang YP, Li L, Shen JZ, Yang FJ, Wu YN. Quinolone-resistance in Salmonella is associated with decreased mRNA expression of virulence genes invA and avrA, growth and intracellular invasion and survival. Vet Microbiol 2009; 133(4): 328-34.
[http://dx.doi.org/10.1016/j.vetmic.2008.07.012] [PMID: 18762392]

[11]   Ferrándiz MJ, Fenoll A, Liñares J, De La Campa AG. Horizontal transfer of parC and gyrA in fluoroquinolone-resistant clinical isolates of *Streptococcus pneumoniae*. Antimicrob Agents Chemother 2000; 44(4): 840-7.
[http://dx.doi.org/10.1128/AAC.44.4.840-847.2000] [PMID: 10722479]

[12]   Hemarajata P, Yang S, Soge OO, Humphries RM, Klausner JD. Performance and verification of a real-time PCR assay targeting the gyrA gene for prediction of ciprofloxacin resistance in Neisseria gonorrhoeae. J Clin Microbiol 2016; 54(3): 805-8.
[http://dx.doi.org/10.1128/JCM.03032-15] [PMID: 26739156]

[13]   Yao C, Zhu T, Li Y, *et al.* Detection of rpoB, katG and inhA gene mutations in Mycobacterium tuberculosis clinical isolates from Chongqing as determined by microarray. Clin Microbiol Infect 2010; 16(11): 1639-43.
[http://dx.doi.org/10.1111/j.1469-0691.2010.03267.x] [PMID: 20491829]

[14]   Loonen AJ, Wolffs PF, Bruggeman CA, van den Brule AJ. Developments for improved diagnosis of bacterial bloodstream infections. Eur J Clin Microbiol Infect Dis 2014; 33(10): 1687-702.
[http://dx.doi.org/10.1007/s10096-014-2153-4] [PMID: 24848132]

[15]   Athamanolap P, Hsieh K, Chen L, Yang S, Wang TH. Integrated bacterial identification and antimicrobial susceptibility testing using PCR and high-resolution melt. Anal Chem 2017; 89(21): 11529-36.
[http://dx.doi.org/10.1021/acs.analchem.7b02809] [PMID: 29027789]

[16]   Koczula KM, Gallotta A. Lateral flow assays. Essays Biochem 2016; 60(1): 111-20.
[http://dx.doi.org/10.1042/EBC20150012] [PMID: 27365041]

[17]   Anjum MF, Mafura M, Slickers P, *et al.* Pathotyping *Escherichia coli* by using miniaturized DNA microarrays. Appl Environ Microbiol 2007; 73(17): 5692-7.
[http://dx.doi.org/10.1128/AEM.00419-07] [PMID: 17630299]

[18]   Zankari E, Hasman H, Cosentino S, *et al.* Identification of acquired antimicrobial resistance genes. J Antimicrob Chemother 2012; 67(11): 2640-4.
[http://dx.doi.org/10.1093/jac/dks261] [PMID: 22782487]

[19]   Palomino JC, Martin A, Von Groll A, Portaels F. Rapid culture-based methods for drug-resistance detection in Mycobacterium tuberculosis. J Microbiol Methods 2008; 75(2): 161-6.
[http://dx.doi.org/10.1016/j.mimet.2008.06.015] [PMID: 18627779]

[20]   Váradi L, Luo JL, Hibbs DE, *et al.* Methods for the detection and identification of pathogenic bacteria: past, present, and future. Chem Soc Rev 2017; 46(16): 4818-32.
[http://dx.doi.org/10.1039/C6CS00693K] [PMID: 28644499]

[21]   Anthony RM, Cobelens FGJ, Gebhard A, *et al.* Liquid culture for Mycobacterium tuberculosis: proceed, but with caution. Int J Tuberc Lung Dis 2009; 13(9): 1051-3.
[PMID: 19723391]

[22]   Jun HJ, Jeon K, Um SW, Kwon OJ, Lee NY, Koh WJ. Nontuberculous mycobacteria isolated during the treatment of pulmonary tuberculosis. Respir Med 2009; 103(12): 1936-40.
[http://dx.doi.org/10.1016/j.rmed.2009.05.025] [PMID: 19576745]

[23]   Ghodbane R, Raoult D, Drancourt M. Dramatic reduction of culture time of Mycobacterium tuberculosis. Sci Rep 2014; 4(1): 4236.
[http://dx.doi.org/10.1038/srep04236] [PMID: 24577292]

[24]   Noster J, Thelen P, Hamprecht A. Detection of multidrug-resistant Enterobacterales—from ESBLs to carbapenemases. Antibiotics (Basel) 2021; 10(9): 1140.
[http://dx.doi.org/10.3390/antibiotics10091140] [PMID: 34572722]

[25]   Shi L, Wu F, Wen Y, Zhao F, Xiang J, Ma L. A novel method to detect Listeria monocytogenes *via* superparamagnetic lateral flow immunoassay. Anal Bioanal Chem 2015; 407(2): 529-35.
[http://dx.doi.org/10.1007/s00216-014-8276-8] [PMID: 25486917]

[26]   Li J, Ma B, Fang J, *et al.* Recombinase polymerase amplification (RPA) combined with lateral flow immunoassay for rapid detection of salmonella in food. Foods 2019; 9(1): 27.
[http://dx.doi.org/10.3390/foods9010027] [PMID: 31887998]

[27]   Zhang Z, Li L, Luo F, *et al.* Rapid and accurate detection of RMP-and INH-resistant Mycobacterium tuberculosis in spinal tuberculosis specimens by CapitalBio™ DNA microarray: A prospective validation study. BMC Infect Dis 2012; 12(1): 1-7.
[http://dx.doi.org/10.1186/1471-2334-12-303]

[28]   Quainoo S, Coolen JPM, van Hijum SAFT, *et al.* Whole-genome sequencing of bacterial pathogens: the future of nosocomial outbreak analysis. Clin Microbiol Rev 2017; 30(4): 1015-63.
[http://dx.doi.org/10.1128/CMR.00016-17] [PMID: 28855266]

[29]   Dlamini MT, Lessells R, Iketleng T, de Oliveira T. Whole genome sequencing for drug-resistant tuberculosis management in South Africa: What gaps would this address and what are the challenges to implementation? J Clin Tuberc Other Mycobact Dis 2019; 16: 100115.
[http://dx.doi.org/10.1016/j.jctube.2019.100115] [PMID: 31720436]

[30]   Frye J G, Lindsey R L, Rondeau G, *et al.* Development of a DNA microarray to detect antimicrobial resistance genes identified in the National Center for Biotechnology Information. Microb Drug Resist 2010; 16(1): 9-19.
[http://dx.doi.org/10.1089/mdr.2009.0082]

CHAPTER 5

Molecular Probes as Diagnostic Tools

Anurag Jyoti[1,*] and **Rajesh Singh Tomar**[1]

[1] *Amity Institute of Biotechnology, Amity University Madhya Pradesh, Maharajpura Dang, Gwalior-474005, M.P., India*

Abstract: Diseases caused by pathogenic microbes have been a serious problem since decades. They often cause high mortality in both developing and developed countries. Diseases including diarrhea, cholera, typhoid, *etc.*, are often involved in outbreaks related to pathogens surviving in water. In recent years, the management of infectious diseases has drawn much attention among scientists and researchers. Various specific, sensitive and reproducible detection methods have been developed to identify pathogen contamination in water. These advanced methods generally use probes for diagnostics of pathogens. The present chapter attempts to focus on the development of various probe chemistries for the detection of pathogens. We also intend to present here the pros and cons of different methods.

Keywords: Amplification, Annealing, Culture, Enumeration, Fluorescence, Infectious disease, Microscopic examination, Molecular Techniques, Mortality, Outbreaks, PCR, Probe, Quantification, Quencher, Real Time PCR, SYBR GREEN1, Sensitivity, Specificity, Template, Target.

INTRODUCTION

Increased population and urbanization have posed challenges to the management of infectious diseases. Water-borne infectious diseases cause major outbreaks in both developing and developed countries. These include diarrhoea, typhoid, cholera and other gastrointestinal diseases [1, 2]. Management of infectious diseases requires several measures. Identification of causative pathogens at the initial level is helpful in the therapeutic regimen of disease. A number of methods exist for the detection of pathogens, including culture-dependent and culture independent methods. All these methods have their own pros and cons. Culture-dependent methods are time consuming and labour intensive. In most laboratory setups, the disease is diagnosed on the basis of microscopic examination of culture. These methods are generally qualitative and, therefore, not applicable for

---

* **Corresponding author Anurag Jyoti:** Amity Institute of Biotechnology, Amity University Madhya Pradesh, Maharajpura Dang, Gwalior-474005, M.P., India; E-mails: ajyoti@gwa.amity.edu, anurag.bt@gmail.com

Sanket Kaushik and Nagendra Singh (Eds.)

disease management. With the span of time, molecular methods have been established and have found their applicability in diagnostics. Polymerase Chain Reaction (PCR) has been established as a standard method for the detection of pathogens. It works on the basis of *in-vitro* amplification of genes or a piece of genes using specific primer pairs. Since this method uses explicit DNA sequences, it is highly specific. Immunological techniques, such as Enzyme Linked Immunosorbent Assay (ELISA), are based on the interaction between antigen-antibody and often get limited due to non-specificity and cross-reactivity.

The development of drug-resistance among causative agents has further complicated the detection system. Various methods, including phenotypic and genotypic methods, are currently used for the quantification of these pathogens. In most of the studies, drug-resistance pattern has been performed using the standard disc-diffusion method using the Clinical Laboratory Standard Institute (CLSI) guidelines, which often give inaccurate results.

Since the last decade, Real Time/Quantitative Polymerase Chain Reaction (RTi-PCR)-based assays have been established as the gold standard in the field of pathogen diagnostics [3, 4]. The method uses molecular probes in addition to the primer pairs. Various probe chemistries are evolved to detect and quantify pathogens present in the sample. The limit of detection (LOD) of this method is very low; therefore, it is used for the diagnostic of pathogens in low doses. Variants of RTi-PCR have revolutionized the quantification of target DNA of pathogenic origin. With the advent of multiplexing, in one assay, enumeration of at least four pathogens can be achieved using different probe chemistries.

Molecular probe-based diagnostics have seen major breakthroughs, and at the same time, they face some challenges. Various methods are there that can reduce the detection time with high sensitivity, including ELISA, Polymerase Chain Reaction (PCR), and so on. Despite improvements, these methods still require more time, sophisticated instrumentation and complex sample preparation steps, which limit their use in diagnostics. In some instances, chances of false positive results occur in DNA amplification-based pathogen detection.

Pathogen detection using molecular probes has revolutionized the management of infectious diseases. The current chapter will provide an overview of the present scenario of molecular probes for pathogen diagnostics.

MOLECULAR DIAGNOSTICS FOR DETECTION OF DRUG-RESISTANT PATHOGENS

Detection of disease-causing pathogens often demands accurate and specific methods. Conventional culture-based methods often face challenges of specificity, sensitivity and rapidity. Classical molecular methods, such as PCR have established themselves in diagnostics. Still, sensitivity and quantification are major hurdles for these techniques and methods. With the advent of RTi-PCR and its various formats, the diagnostics of pathogens have been revolutionized, saving time with improved sensitivity and ease of quantification. Various probe chemistries have been used in RTi-PCR based diagnosis of pathogens.

Detection of drug-resistant pathogens is a real challenging task. Advancements of genome sequencing and identification of genes, responsible for drug-resistance and virulence has opened new avenue towards detection of these pathogens. The development of duplex PCR-based system has shown the potential to detect pathogens in low doses. Detection of virulent gene and drug-resistant genes simultaneously in single tube format gives quick results for the identification of pathogens.

Polymerase Chain Reactions (PCR)

PCR is one of the most important disruptive technologies in molecular biology. DNA molecules are amplified in *in-vitro* conditions using specific primer pairs. Each round of PCR produces new double stranded DNA molecules. Primer pairs are designed using dedicated software to ensure specificity. Certain portions of DNA of the pathogen of interest are targeted and primers are designed accordingly. PCR consists of 3 major steps: Denaturation, Annealing and Extension. During denaturation, the double stranded (ds) DNA gets separated and will serve as templates for primers, while in annealing, the temperature is lowered down and both the primers and the DNA templates get aligned themselves at their respective complementary strands. During extension, each primer pair extends and generates a new pair of double stranded DNA. Two important factors impact the pathogen detection using PCR: a) Selection of conserved regions of genes, unique to the target organism and b) Optimization of annealing temperature for complete binding of primer pair with respective DNA template.

A number of studies exist that use PCR for the detection of pathogens. This includes pathogens causing diseases in plants, animals and human beings. Mirmajlessi *et al.* (2015) has presented review on detection of pathogens on strawberry using PCR [5]. Stockmann *et al.* (2015) has compared standard microbiologic testing with the multiplex polymerase chain reaction (PCR) system that simultaneously detects 23 diarrhoeal pathogens [6].

Real Time Polymerase Chain Reactions (PCR)

Real time PCR is an advanced assay for sensitive quantification of amplifiable DNA sequences. In addition to the oligonucleotide primer pair, the assay uses oligonucleotide probes. These molecular probes enhance the specificity and sensitivity of the assay. Various probe chemistries are there for the quantification of target DNA. RTi-PCR is based on the application of fluorescent labelled probes to identify and quantify the amplicons. The assay is fast compared to conventional PCR, as there is no need for post-PCR analysis on agarose gel. RTi-PCR works on the principle of generation of fluorescence when PCR products are generated. Initial signal is generated in the first 40-50 minutes, depending upon the amount of target present. The complete assay is performed in a closed tube system; therefore, there is no cross-over contamination and chances of false positive and false negative are minimized. In RTi-PCR, amplification and quantification of the target DNA are monitored simultaneously. The RTi-PCR thermal cycler is equipped with software that records the fluorescence and displays it in relative fluorescence units (RFU). The cycle at which a significant fluorescence is recorded exceeding the basal cut-off level is known as the cycle threshold (C_T). A higher amount of template DNA will certainly reach the cycle threshold earlier as more fluorescence is produced with respect to amplification.

Detection Chemistries

The fluorescent reporters can be classified on the basis of nucleic acid dyes and molecular probes.

Nucleic Acid Dye: SYBR Green I

SYBR Green I is a fluorescence-based dye that binds non-specifically to any double-stranded DNA. The resulting DNA-dye-complex absorption (λ_{max} = 498 nm) and emission maxima (λ_{max} = 522 nm). SYBR Green, in its bound state, emits a strong fluorescent signal (depending on the amount of amplicon), which can be discriminated from that emitted by unbound dye. The ease of use of SYBR Green in DNA detection makes it advantageous over other methods. Apart from this, lower cost, computation-free designing of assays makes SYBR Green as a preferred choice in RTi-PCR based detection formats. As the fluorophore is non-specific towards dsDNA, it can bind to any dsDNA. This often leads to the generation of false positive signals. The SYBR Green based assay has an additional feature of melt curve analysis. The melting curve analysis is performed just after amplification. This additional feature allows exposing the amplicons with high temperature and the fluorescence is recorded. Analysis of the melting curve provides the user to make a distinction between desired amplicons and non-specific amplicons. SYBR Green I has been applied successfully in real time PCR (McCrea *et al.* 2007). *Escherichia coli* O157:H7, *Listeria monocytogenes*, and *Salmonella* strains in fresh produce have been detected simultaneously using SYBR Green I and melting curve analysis [7].

Sequence-specific Probe

Molecular Beacon (MB)

Molecular beacon is a small (25-35 bases long), single stranded oligonucleotide molecule that forms a hairpin with loop and self-complementary stem. The loop, anactual probe, is computed to hybridize to a specific region of the target DNA sequence. Stems are self-complementary, and often constitute 5-7 bases. At both the ends (5' and 3' ends) of MB probe, fluorophore molecules are attached. The emission maxima of fluorophore attached at 5'end overlaps with the excitation maxima of fluorophore attached at the 3'end. The fluorescent reporter molecule attached at 5'-end gives fluorescence, when MB probe binds with the target. In its unbound state with the target sequence, the MB probe exists in closed hair-pin loop structure. Therefore, the emitted fluorescence by fluorophore at 5'-end will be quenched by quencher at 3'end and no signal is generated. During the annealing step of the amplification reaction, the MB probe binds to the respective target; as a result both the fluorophore and quencher are distant apart and contact-dependent quenching cannot be achieved. As a result, the fluorescence is recorded, which corresponds to amplification of the target DNA [8]. MB probe has a high degree of specificity and sensitivity towards target detection. Moreover, there is no need for melt-curve analysis. The probe has been used to detect a number of pathogens [9, 10].

CONCLUSION

The management of drug-resistant infectious diseases is often limited by the availability of accurate and sensitive diagnostic tools. Molecular technology-based diagnostic methods show unmatched potential for the detection and quantification of pathogens in low doses. Various probe chemistries enhance the rapidity, specificity and sensitivity of the detection system. Multiplexing in probe-based quantitative Polymerase Chain Reaction has revolutionized the detection of multiple pathogens in a single assay. Drug-resistant genes are targeted for the detection of pathogens. Although the probe-based chemistries have potential to detect drug-resistant pathogens, still they have some shortcomings. False positives/negatives, the requirement of trained personnel, expensive reagents, *etc.*, often limit the applicability of these methods.

CONSENT FOR PUBLICATION

Not applicable.

CONFLICT OF INTEREST

The authors declare no conflict of interest, financial or otherwise.

ACKNOWLEDGEMENTS

The authors wish to express our sincere acknowledgment to Dr. Ashok Kumar Chauhan, President, RBEF parent organization of Amity University Madhya Pradesh (AUMP), Dr. Aseem Chauhan, Additional President, RBEF and Chancellor, AUMP, Gwalior, Lt. Gen. V.K. Sharma, AVSM (Retd.), Vice Chancellor of AUMP, Gwalior for providing facilities, their Valuable support and encouragement throughout the work.

REFERENCES

[1]   Tomar RS, Jyoti A. Culture-independent quantification of Salmonellae in food by molecular beacon based real-time PCR. J Appl Pharm Sci 2016; 6: 153-7.
        [http://dx.doi.org/10.7324/JAPS.2016.601124]

[2]   Jyoti A, Tomar RS. Detection of pathogenic bacteria using nanobiosensors. Environ Chem Lett 2016; 1-6.

[3]   Ram S, Vajpayee P, Shanker R. Rapid culture-independent quantitative detection of enterotoxigenic *Escherichia coli* in surface waters by real-time PCR with molecular beacon. Environ Sci Technol 2008; 42(12): 4577-82.
        [http://dx.doi.org/10.1021/es703033u] [PMID: 18605589]

[4]   Jyoti A, Vajpayee P, Singh G, Patel CB, Gupta KC, Shanker R. Identification of environmental reservoirs of nontyphoidal salmonellosis: aptamer-assisted bioconcentration and subsequent detection of *salmonella typhimurium* by quantitative polymerase chain reaction. Environ Sci Technol 2011; 45(20): 8996-9002.
        [http://dx.doi.org/10.1021/es2018994] [PMID: 21875107]

[5]   Mirmajlessi SM, Destefanis M, Gottsberger RA, Mänd M, Loit E. PCR-based specific techniques used for detecting the most important pathogens on strawberry: a systematic review. Syst Rev 2015; 4: 9.
        [http://dx.doi.org/10.1186/2046-4053-4-9] [PMID: 25588564]

[6]   Stockmann C, Rogatcheva M, Harrel B, *et al.* How well does physician selection of microbiologic tests identify *Clostridium difficile* and other pathogens in paediatric diarrhoea? Insights using multiplex PCR-based detection. Clin Microbiol Infect 2015; 21(2): 179.e9-179.e15.
        [http://dx.doi.org/10.1016/j.cmi.2014.07.011] [PMID: 25599941]

[7]   McCrea JK, Liu C, Ng LK, Wang G. Detection of the Escherichia coli pathogenic gene eae with three real-time polymerase chain reaction methods. Can J Microbiol 2007; 53(3): 398-403.
        [http://dx.doi.org/10.1139/W06-148] [PMID: 17538649]

[8]   Bhagwat AA. Simultaneous detection of *Escherichia coli* O157:H7, *Listeria monocytogenes* and Salmonella strains by real-time PCR. Int J Food Microbiol 2003; 84(2): 217-24.
        [http://dx.doi.org/10.1016/S0168-1605(02)00481-6] [PMID: 12781944]

[9]   Tyagi S, Kramer FR. Molecular beacons in diagnostics. F1000 Med Rep 2012; 4: 10.
        [http://dx.doi.org/10.3410/M4-10] [PMID: 22619695]

[10]   Chavda KD, Satlin M, Chen L, *et al.* Evaluation of a Multiplex PCR Assay with Molecular Beacon Probes to Rapidly Detect Bacterial Pathogens Directly in Bronchial Alveolar Lavage (BAL) Samples from Patients with Hospital-Acquired Pneumonia (HAP). Open Forum Infect Dis 2017; 4 (Suppl. 1): S614.
[http://dx.doi.org/10.1093/ofid/ofx163.1616]

CHAPTER 6

Real-Time PCR High-Resolution Melting Analysis

Ena Gupta[1], Sanket Kaushik[1], Vijay Kumar Srivastava[1], Juhi Saxena[2] and Anupam Jyoti[2,*]

[1] *Amity Institute of Biotechnology, Amity University Rajasthan, Amity Education Valley, Kant Kalwar, NH-11C, Jaipur-Delhi Highway, Jaipur, India*

[2] *Department of Biotechnology, University Institute of Biotechnology, Chandigarh University, Mohali, Punjab, 140413, India*

Abstract: High Resolution Melting (HRM) is a homogeneous, exceptionally incredible innovation for single nucleotide polymorphism (SNP) genotyping, mutation scanning and sequence scanning in DNA samples. HRM analysis works on the principle of melting (dissociation) curve methodologies of Polymerase Chain Reaction (PCR) empowered by the new accessibility of improved double-stranded DNA (dsDNA)–binding dyes and next-generation real-time PCR instrumentation. The HRM technology portrays samples of nucleic acids on the basis of their disassociation behaviors and identifies the differences in even the short sequence in amplified PCR products, just by direct melting. Samples are further distinguished according to the length of their sequence, GC content and strand complementarity. Indeed, even a single change in the base pair in the sequences of DNA samples causes differences in the HRM curve. The difference in the melting curves of different genetic sequences at distinct rates can be observed, detected and compared using these curves. Development of the melting curves after HRM analysis is basically plotted with temperature on the X axis and fluorescence on the Y axis, which resembles the real-time PCR amplification curve but with the difference of temperature for cycle number. With the use of different DNA dyes, high-end instrumentation and sophisticated analysis software, these distinctions are detected.

Keywords: Antimicrobial resistance, Genotyping, Genetic variants, HRMA, Intercalating dyes, Melting curve.

INTRODUCTION

Because of the high demand for brisk, highly-throughput examination and genetic study of microbes in addition to data handling and research, focus should be on

* **Corresponding author Anupam Jyoti:** Department of Biotechnology, University Institute of Biotechnology, Chandigarh University, Mohali, Punjab, 140413, India;
E-mail: anupam.e12214@cumail.in

the significant interpretation and improvement of advanced mechanism of detection that counteracts the requirement for electrophoretic analysis, decrease the exposure of contamination and significantly reduce labor time and reagent expenses [1]. Thus, new advances in methods, instruments, fluorescent dyes and different operating systems for melting analysis of DNA have devised a more flexible novel technique for an alternative scanning and genotyping, *i.e.*, a comparatively novel approach of post-PCR analysis allowing the analysis of characterization of PCR amplicons in a closed structure [2].

Earlier analysis of the melting curves of PCR product together along-with real-time was recommended with the Light Cyclers [3]. No processing or separations were required like many DNA analysis methods. The DNA duplexes resistance was scanned as the temperature was increased in the solution by the fluorescence of SYBRs Green I. Even though large variation in PCR products was differentiated by melting temperature (Tm), refined sequence fluctuations were considered beyond the reach of fluorescent melting analysis. HRMA (high resolution DNA melting) was initially reported in 2002, and it has since been widely utilised as a research tool [4] and as a quick approach for genotyping known variations or scanning for undiscovered variants [5].

HRMA is logical, economical and rapid approach that requires labelled probes. The sensitivity of heterozygote scanning reaches 100% with the expansion of saturating dye prior to PCR and rapid melting curve analysis of the amplicons. To reduce the burden of sequencing, researchers might examine common heterogeneity with the melting of shorter amplicons and unlabeled probes. Different heterozygotes create comparable melting curves, but unlike homozygous variants, they do not discriminate [2].

For discerning variances and heterogeneity in nucleic acid sequencing, HRM analysis is a more sophisticated, inventive, robust, and closed-tube, high-throughput method [6, 7]. HRM allows for the discovery of genetic variants by analysing PCR melting curves of DNA with spectacular temperature resolution while using a saturating DNA-binding dye of high grade and advanced instrumentation software [6]. Its procedures also create unique and sensitive melting profiles, which may be used in genotyping, mutation screening, and methylation studies using heterozygozygosity, length, and GC content [8]. HRM utilizes cheap dyes and needs low optimization that works on similar platforms like TaqMan along with fluorescence resonance energy transfer (FRET) probes. HRM, on comparison to such approaches, gives better results as it is uncomplicated, coherent and more economical way to characterize more than one sample. HRMA is an elementary PCR that lacks the necessity for any big alterations in the laboratory with any specific skills. It performs under customized conditions in a close vicinity of a specific dye. The most expensive element is the recovery of the instrument [9].

To some extent, HRM is a recent post-PCR approach that analyses the shape of the melting curve followed by amplification of PCR with saturating DNA dye, resulting in a specific amplicon melting curve, allowing the detection of small sequence variants. The present technique is obsolete used effectively for mutation scanning, SNPs genotyping, and identifying several bacterial species, as well as screening for drug resistance in pathogens [10 - 12]. Besides genotyping, HRM real-time PCR has been revealed to have an interesting capability of SNP identification across the genes which are involved in drug resistance [13]. Many researches have demonstrated HRM real-time PCR for the identification of mutations associated with drug resistance throughout the last decade. Resistant to antibiotics is assessed by utilizing culture based techniques *i.e.* the agar percentage methods or liquid media methods such as the BACTEC MGIT 960. However, these approaches are not efficient and need therapeutic susceptibility testing which takes at least a week, as they are effective [14]. It is clinically critical for patients to have an early drug susceptibility result in order to begin an appropriate therapeutic regimen that will result in improved outcomes. It also enables the monitoring of antibiotic resistance rates, which are important in the fight against infection [15].

PRINCIPLE OF THE MELTING PROFILE

Various intercalating dyes are utilized by the Post-PCR melt curve analysis to identify primer-dimmers or any other non-specific products. This process is known as Low Resolution Melting. While the temperature rises, a curve is generated in increments with 0.5 °C, thus constantly denaturing of an amplified DNA target. The dye used is primarily fluorescent, but when the duplex DNA is denatured, the fluorescence gradually decreases when attached to dsDNA. The length, GC content, sequencing, and heterozygosity of the amplified target all influence the melting profile [16].

At the melting temperature of a DNA sample, the highest rate of fluorescence declination is usually measured. As a result, the temperature at which half of a DNA sample is double stranded and the other half is single stranded is known as the Tm temperature. For fragmented DNA that is longer and/or has a higher GC content, the Tm temperature is generally greater [17]. By analyzing the curve of fluorescence *vs.* Temperature (-dF/dT versus T), data from weak fluorescence resolution melting curves may be utilised to determine the temperature (Fig. **1**).

Rise in the temperature during a low-resolution melt curve analysis is in 0.5 °C steps and this is reduced to 0.008 - 0.2 °C increments for HRM analysis. That is why the principle of HRM works on the same principle of low-resolution melt. This permits more specific observations of the melting performance [18].

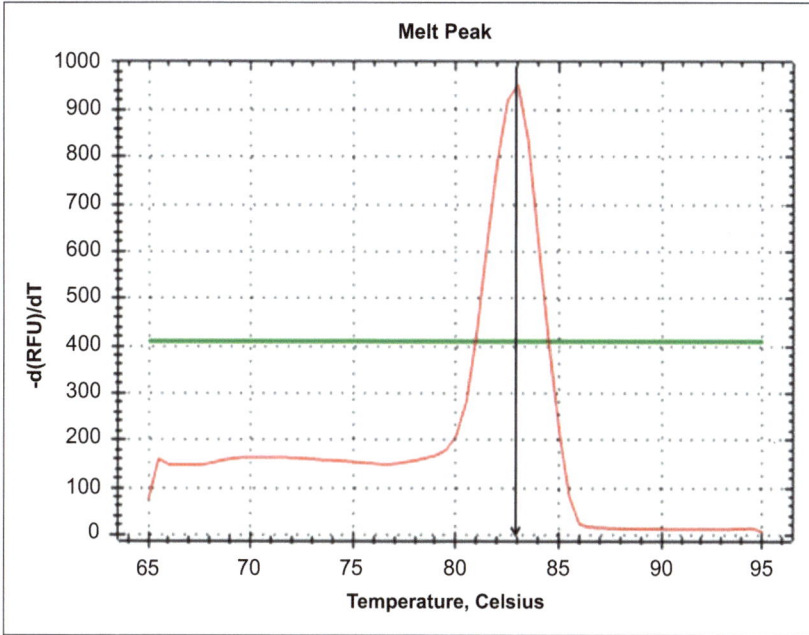

Fig. (1). The steepest slope is easily visualized as a melting peak where the Tm of the amplicon is 83 °C.

INTERCALATING DYES

Several types of dsDNA intercalating dyes are present with individual characteristics that provide extensive information on an amplified target's melting efficiency. Due to the change in the melting temperature of the amplicon or inhibition in the amplification of DNA, dye should not bind to purines or pyrimidines. Intercalating dyes are engaged to pursue the change of dsDNA to ssDNA. Depending on the cooperation, these dyes show differential fluorescence emission with dsDNA or ss DNA [19].

Non-saturating Dyes

SYBR Green I is the utmost frequently used non saturating first generation double stranded DNA intercalating dye for HRM that fluoresces when intercalated only with dsDNA and not ssDNA. However, it is incompatible with many HRM applications since greater concentrations may inhibit PCR, stabilise duplex DNA, and inhibit DNA polymerase, necessitating the use of smaller concentrations. It has the capacity to redistribute melted ssDNA segments back to dsDNA regions at lower concentrations, resulting in poor base difference discrimination. Some researchers have denied the use of SYBR Green I for HRM, insisting some significant modifications in the protocol are needed due to the lack of accuracy resulting from "dye jumping", in which the dye from a melted duplex may get integrated into different targets of dsDNA which is still not yet melted [20]. Saturating dyes, the best examples to overcome this drawback, have been developed [21].

Saturating Dyes

Recently developed novel advance class of intercalating dyes that do not alter the Tm of the product or inhibit the DNA polymerases. These dyes are applied at high concentrations compared to non saturating dyes, resulting in complete intercalation of the amplicon. This dye is unable to disperse after melting because the double stranded DNA is saturated. At the saturating concentrations necessary for HRM, dyes like SYTO9 and LCGreen can be utilized [22].

Release-on-demand Dyes

These dyes are added at non-saturating concentrations including Eva Green dyes. The dye is freely available in the solution where the fluorescent signal is quenched. This is the innovative method used for fluorescence emission. When the quenching factor is released, the dye emits high fluorescent signal on binding to dsDNA. This permits the requirement of the concentration of non saturating dyes which provide no PCR inhibition; also, the chemistry of this rare dye administers highly sensitive analysis of HRM [23].

WORKING OF PCR-HRM

Since various dyes have distinct emission spectra, proper calibration of the instrument prior to usage is critical. For the correct calibration of the instrument proper adjustment is essential for each set of reagents. The demand for proper design of assay for successful HRM analysis is very much critical. Correct primer selection, DNA quality, reagent selection, and protocol optimization are all key factors in attaining the best possible results. If an assay has previously been optimised, the PCR may be done on any normal thermo-cycler, and then the samples are transferred to a real-time thermo-cycler that can conduct HRM after the last PCR cycle. Many distinct settings are usually necessary to manage the instrument, which combines the start and end temperatures, as well as the rise in temperature calculating the hold durations between data recovery, which are typically 0.008 – 0.2 °C steps with a 2 second hold-time. As a result, few equipments never permit a higher level of elasticity and instead use a single protocol that cannot be altered [24 - 27].

Analysis of Data

With innovative, resilient, and sophisticated software tools, several specimens may be analyzed at the same time, with data analysis that is typically accurate and straightforward. While analyzing the melting profiles of raw HRM, it is critical to know and understand what to seek.

As shown in Fig. (**2A**), Fluorescence readings were taken across a wide range of temperatures and separated into three parts: pre-melt, melt, and post-melt, in the raw data produced during the HRM analysis. Despite the fact that the different genotype groups are readily evident, the fluctuations make it much more important to evaluate the data. The parallel double-bars inside the interface must be placed with which the data is normalised to choose pre- and post-melt zones. If the pre- or post-melt zones are unable to be accurately examined, the HRM run should be resumed with the appropriate range of temperature [28, 29].

Only when the range of temperature is shown between the outer bars of the pre- and post-melt region and the fluorescence difference is removed from the pre- or post-melt regions, then this type of plot is known as "Normalization Data." In this type of data, the genotypes are now more specific, but the change in melting curves is usually small in some cases [30]. If the data is correctly analyzed, the "normalized" data will emerge, as shown in Fig. (**2B**).

Some software applications of HRM allow the calculation of a yielding curve to analyze small deference's better between the specific melting curves of the amplicons, which is done when the normalized fluorescence data of a user-defined genotype is subtracted from that of each of the specimens within the period of HRM analysis. In Fig. (**2C**), the position of every sample is plotted against the temperature, which is absolutely helpful for visualizing the normalization data of HRM [31, 32].

Factors Affecting HRM

Care should be taken for productive examination to validate that the performance of the experiment is enhanced correctly for HRM. Although priority should be given to the designing of primers along with the PCR reagents and cycling conditions. Because only minor changes in melting curves may be induced by factors other than the nucleotide sequence, achieving selective amplification is critical to the HRM assay's efficiency, as any non-specific amplification would significantly hinder the melt analysis [33, 34].

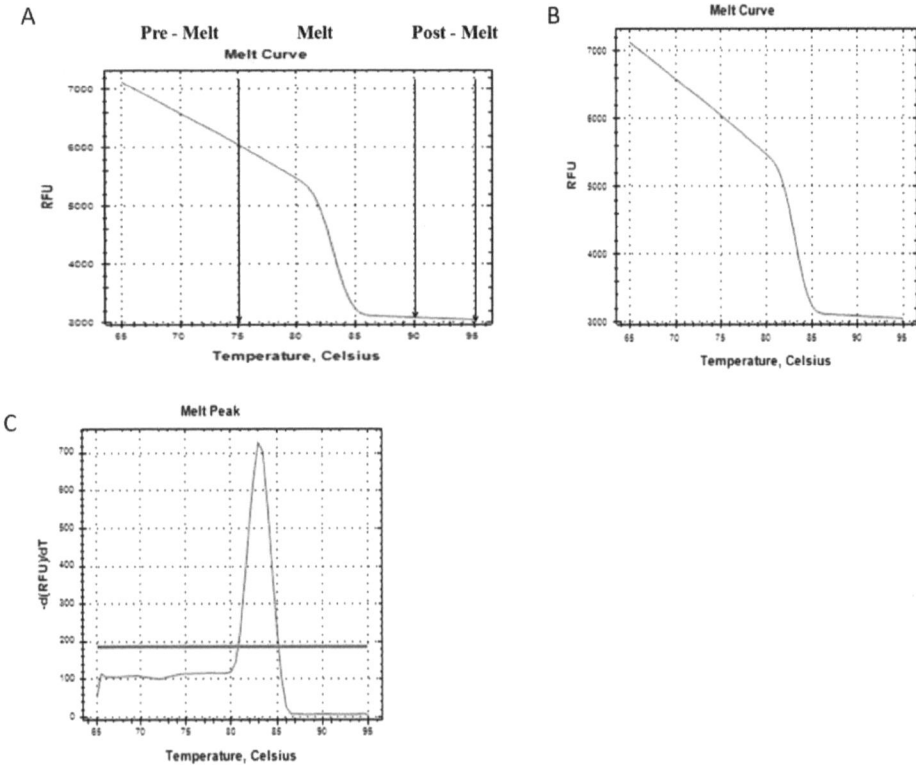

Fig. (2). A). Raw data showing the pre-melt, melt and post-melt regions. **B).** Normalization Data is derived from the basic data plots in A. **C).** Difference Graph attained from the normalization data.

Many such factors of the genomic DNA (gDNA) such as quality, length of the amplicon, design of the primer, selection of the dye and PCR settings will all hinder the melting behavior; for example; a DNA template with lower quality may develop non-specific products of PCR resulting in lower sensitivity or failed experiments with false genotype. An incomplete or low-resolution HRM data is detected for the late amplified samples or declined to achieve a higher signal peak in the PCR phase. In an analysis, all the DNA specimens must be processed using the similar methodology for the most effective and positive results. For the same threshold cycle (Ct) values, the concentrations of the DNA samples should not differ too much [35, 36].

Moreover, whenever possible immediately after the PCR, HRM analysis should be achieved and usually the length of an amplicon is suggested at 50–300 bp for best since the length plays a major role, it becomes more challenging to distinguish between sequence variations, HRM analysis of unique sequence variants such as SNPs, insertions, inversions, and deletions was performed. When screening for distinguishing unknown sequences, however, amplicons of a length of 200–500 bp are considered [33, 37]. This helps in scanning gene or examining the deviation in a population. Primers designing should be enhanced on a priority basis because of the intercalation of the dyes to any dsDNA products for robust performance and specificity to the region of interest. In addition, in the case of the same melting profiles, the HRM software is incapable of detecting non-specific reaction products. So, it is just better to initially evaluate PCR amplicons by agarose gel electrophoresis [2].

The quality of the PCR conditions is further essential factor along with the variety of intercalating dye as a distinct variety of HRM dyes should be approved before identifying which dye functions best, in a given experimental system. The PCR parameters should be modified to produce appropriate amplification, which is driven by decreased Ct-values and amplification curves [36]. Because various instruments utilise different detection methods, another important factor impacting dye functionality is the instrument itself.

APPLICATIONS

The ability to differentiate individual copies of numerous nucleic acid targets of interest in a heterogeneous sample is a crucial difficulty in clinical diagnostic development and basic bimolecular research [38 - 43]. However, HRM technique is robust, advanced, attractive, and cost-effective SNP genotyping technology that rely on the examination of the melting profile of PCR. Following are some of the notable applications of HRM technology [42, 43].

Identification of Microbial Species

To identify the microbial species, HRM analysis of housekeeping genes or other highly conserved genes is obsoletely utilized widely. Species identification in *Mycobacterium chelonae*, *M. abscessus* group were first reported applications of HRM [44]. No universal HRM-based technology has been claimed for pathogen identification, which are mainly focusing upon particular genera with published methods [45], specific on the classes of bio-threat agent species [46], or particular class of species that are coherent to be detected in sepsis [47]. HRM analysis was used to differentiate between *Cryptococcus grubii*, *C. neoformans*, and *C. gattii* species by investigating a 100bp fragment of internal transcribed spacer 1 from ribosomal DNA [48]. The detailed diagnosis and description from culture as well as tissue samples of muco-mycetes have undeniable brisk utilization in the diagnostic field [49].

Mutation Detection

For the identification of variants of DNA sequence, HRMA has been developed and it was first practiced for genotyping [5]. Simple, economical, and easy to use with increased specificity and sensitivity are some eminent features that make HRMA more attractive and a novel technique applied in diagnostic labs for genotyping [50].

Marcin Słomka (2017) validates the HRM technology as a practical approach for scanning genes as well as genotyping single and multiple SNPs. To scan for both quantitative analysis (deletions/duplications) as well as qualitative analysis of the nucleotide changes in one assay, Lasa-Fernandez (2020) observed the quantitative PCR and HRMA simultaneously in one instrument [51]. Also, S Chakraborty *et al*. (2019) characterized the utilization of HRMA for scanning the whole genome for sequence variants [52]. Since many of them are hetero-plasmic with the variant allele, the identification of variants is very much complicated as they are present at highly variable percentages. There is evidence that scientists have favorably determined the variants with 1–100% of heteroplasmy, which accurately demonstrated the sensitivity, including the potency of HRMA to detect quantitative changes [53].

Microbial Genotyping within Species

Presently, there is a need of high-throughput and inexpensive methodologies like molecular typing for the tracking of epidemiological episodes along with monitoring of microorganisms. Single-locus sequence typing method was a widely used typing method, which works on hyper variable gene fragments. HRM may resolve substantial numbers of alleles of single loci, as demonstrated by the research of fowl adenovirus, which demonstrates the value of HRM analysis of an unusually wide region of base pair that creates HRM curves routinely with many melting domains [54]. Methods such as Multi-locus HRM-based microbial genotyping with higher resolving power have also been developed for the investigation of recombine-genic species with imperfect allelic linkage.

An innovative use of HRM technology has been devised to figure out the variety of HIV in a certain host [55]. When duplexes melt in a sample inside an amplicon, the increased variety of sequence variation emerges throughout a larger temperature range, as assessed by the breadth of the dF/dT curve [56].

Identification of Genotypic Variants Leading to Antimicrobial Resistance

Leading to antimicrobial resistance, detection of genotypic variants is now possible by the HRM analysis. HRM is utilized to diagnose variants and specific SNPs in a particular gene correlated with antimicrobial resistance where phenotypic assays for AMR are very critical to achieve.

The fact that phenotypic testing takes several weeks is a significant obstacle to using resistance testing in a timely manner. Various drugs are taken into practice for the treatment of specific mutation pathways leading to resistance. As Compared to phenotypic susceptibility testing, the current study targets regions for examination by HRM, which is found in the ranges of sensitivity and specificity of 94% to 100% and 98% to 100% to identify resistance [57]. The evolution of false negatives was caused by resistance mutations occurring beyond the targeted areas, whereas false positives were caused by the diagnosis of similar mutations. However, sophisticated and compelling properties of this assay, such as its low cost and speed, make it an attractive technique of screening for gene changes linked to drug resistance.

Identification of Human Genetic Variants of Importance to Susceptibility to or Treatment of Infectious Diseases

The discovery of human gene variations that discuss the vulnerability of infectious diseases is critical. These are critical for the host's reaction to therapy, and they are the future use of HRM analysis. The collaboration of the polymorphism in the interleukin gene based on the interferon response with medicines for chronic hepatitis C virus infections is an outstanding example. HRM analysis of the 59-bp region clearly discriminated the CC, TT, and CT variants with 100% concordance to sequencing [58].

Alternative for Gel Electrophoresis

Current standard to check the result of a PCR product or digestion is analyzed by using agarose gel electrophoresis and ethidium–bromide staining. Since the characterization of each fragment is identified by its length, purity by the absence of any foreign fragments and production by the energy of the fluorescence of the band. HRMA is an interesting substitute and its integrity is characterized by the melting profile, purity is checked by the absence of deformity from the control melt curve or the absence of any further melt peaks, and output is confirmed by the quantity of fluorescence signal. The advantages of utilizing the advanced technique HRMA is very much prompt and accurate as user does not have to pour gels and use harmful chemicals (ethidium–bromide) is not required, melting is rapid than electrophoresis, and data analysis can be interpreted automatically [30].

CONCLUSION

The convenient aspect of HRMA causes this technology to quickly fascinate a range of new users. Comfortable to use, simple, flexible, economical, nondestructive nature, superb sensitivity and specificity make this methodology a preference to scan patients for microbial variants. HRMA has many novel applications, making this a flexible multipurpose analytical tool to diagnose and identify nucleic acids. Still, HRMA is a relatively novel methodology; future advances can only be fascinating and amazing [59]. Although this approach has not been widely adopted, particularly in clinical practice, several characteristics such as higher sensitivity, flexibility, and being economical render it a viable tool for infectious disease screening by reducing the risk of false negative results by systematically monitoring the yields of DNA extraction and the potential interference of PCR inhibitors in each run and for all samples, especially in endemic regions. To establish PCR- HRM efficacy as a diagnostic tool, larger prospective multicentric studies investigating multiple types of samples (clinical) are required [60]. Future studies will focus on enhancing DNA quality and directly applying HRM to different medications and clinical specimens to improve HRM efficacy for detecting drug-resistant mutations. Drug sensitivity analysis based on gene identification will be enhanced in the future, and HRM will be more optimal, thanks to a better knowledge of drug resistance mechanisms [61]. Furthermore, it appears that HRM real-time PCR's capabilities for simultaneous detection and genotyping, as well as assessment of infection load and presence of resistance genes, can give a wealth of information in clinical and epidemiological research [62].

CONSENT FOR PUBLICATION

Not applicable.

CONFLICT OF INTEREST

The authors declare no conflict of interest, financial or otherwise.

ACKNOWLEDGEMENTS

We are indebted to the Indian Council of Medical Research, New Delhi, India (2019-5517/CMB-BMS), for providing financial support. We also acknowledge Amity University Rajasthan, Jaipur, Chandigarh University, Mohali for offering their important help, support and encouragement all through the work.

REFERENCES

[1]   Ngui R, Lim YA, Chua KH. Rapid detection and identification of human hookworm infections through high resolution melting (HRM) analysis. PLoS One 2012; 7(7): e41996.
[http://dx.doi.org/10.1371/journal.pone.0041996] [PMID: 22844538]

[2]   Li M, Zhou L, Palais RA, Wittwer CT. Genotyping accuracy of high-resolution DNA melting instruments. Clin Chem 2014; 60(6): 864-72.
[http://dx.doi.org/10.1373/clinchem.2013.220160] [PMID: 24718912]

[3]   Erali M, Wittwer CT. High resolution melting analysis for gene scanning. Methods 2010; 50(4): 250-61.
[http://dx.doi.org/10.1016/j.ymeth.2010.01.013] [PMID: 20085814]

[4]   Ruskova L, Raclavsky V. The potential of high-resolution melting analysis (hrma) to streamline, facilitate and enrich routine diagnostics in medical microbiology. Biomedical Papers of the Medical Faculty of Palacky University in Olomouc 2011.

[5]   Hwang IT. Cyclic-CMTA: an innovative concept in multiplex quantification. Seegene Bulletin 2012; 1: 11-5.

[6]   Ebili H, Ilyas M. High resolution melt analysis, DNA template quantity disparities and result reliability. Clin Lab 2015; 61(1-2): 155-9.
[http://dx.doi.org/10.7754/Clin.Lab.2014.140821] [PMID: 25807649]

[7]   Tong SY, Giffard PM. Microbiological applications of high-resolution melting analysis. J Clin Microbiol 2012; 50(11): 3418-21.
[http://dx.doi.org/10.1128/JCM.01709-12] [PMID: 22875887]

[8]   Lochlainn SÓ, Amoah S, Graham NS, *et al.* High Resolution Melt (HRM) analysis is an efficient tool to genotype EMS mutants in complex crop genomes. Plant Methods 2011; 7(1): 43.
[http://dx.doi.org/10.1186/1746-4811-7-43] [PMID: 22152063]

[9]   Druml B, Cichna-Markl M. High resolution melting (HRM) analysis of DNA--its role and potential in food analysis. Food Chem 2014; 158: 245-54.
[http://dx.doi.org/10.1016/j.foodchem.2014.02.111] [PMID: 24731338]

[10]   Ramirez MV, Cowart KC, Campbell PJ, *et al.* Rapid detection of multidrug-resistant *Mycobacterium tuberculosis* by use of real-time PCR and high-resolution melt analysis. J Clin Microbiol 2010; 48(11): 4003-9.
[http://dx.doi.org/10.1128/JCM.00812-10] [PMID: 20810777]

[11]   Pang Y, Liu G, Wang Y, Zheng S, Zhao YL. Combining COLD-PCR and high-resolution melt analysis for rapid detection of low-level, rifampin-resistant mutations in *Mycobacterium tuberculosis.* J Microbiol Methods 2013; 93(1): 32-6.
[http://dx.doi.org/10.1016/j.mimet.2013.01.008] [PMID: 23396215]

[12]   Krypuy M, Ahmed AA, Etemadmoghadam D, *et al.* High resolution melting for mutation scanning of TP53 exons 5-8. BMC Cancer 2007; 7(1): 168.
[http://dx.doi.org/10.1186/1471-2407-7-168] [PMID: 17764544]

[13]   Liu FW, Ding ST, Lin EC, Lu YW, Jang JSR. Automated melting curve analysis in droplet microfluidics for single nucleotide polymorphisms (SNP) genotyping. RSC Advances 2017; 7(8): 4646-55.
[http://dx.doi.org/10.1039/C6RA26484K]

[14]   Telles MA, Bori A, Amorim AB, Cruz AF, Pini MI, Sato DN. Rapid detection of multidrug-resistant *Mycobacterium tuberculosis* using the mycobacteria growth indicator tube (MGIT) system. Braz J Med Biol Res 2002; 35(10): 1127-31.
[http://dx.doi.org/10.1590/S0100-879X2002001000003] [PMID: 12424483]

[15]   Bozeman L, Burman W, Metchock B, Welch L, Weiner M. Fluoroquinolone susceptibility among *Mycobacterium tuberculosis* isolates from the United States and Canada. Clin Infect Dis 2005; 40(3):

386-91.
[http://dx.doi.org/10.1086/427292] [PMID: 15668861]

[16] Sarkinfada F, Auwal I, Manu AY. Applications of molecular diagnostic techniques for infectious diseases. Bayero J Pure Appl Sci 2014; 7(1): 37-45.
[http://dx.doi.org/10.4314/bajopas.v7i1.8]

[17] Auwal IK. Nucleic Acid Amplification as used in the Diagnosis and Management of Viral Diseases: A Review. Bayero J Pure Appl Sci 2014; 7(1): 24-33.
[http://dx.doi.org/10.4314/bajopas.v7i1.6]

[18] Zhou L, Palais RA, Paxton CN, Geiersbach KB, Wittwer CT. Copy number assessment by competitive PCR with limiting deoxynucleotide triphosphates and high-resolution melting. Clin Chem 2015; 61(5): 724-33.
[http://dx.doi.org/10.1373/clinchem.2014.236208] [PMID: 25759466]

[19] Ihle MA, Fassunke J, König K, *et al.* Comparison of high resolution melting analysis, pyrosequencing, next generation sequencing and immunohistochemistry to conventional Sanger sequencing for the detection of p.V600E and non-p.V600E BRAF mutations. BMC Cancer 2014; 14(1): 13.
[http://dx.doi.org/10.1186/1471-2407-14-13] [PMID: 24410877]

[20] Miyaoka Y, Berman JR, Cooper SB, *et al.* Systematic quantification of HDR and NHEJ reveals effects of locus, nuclease, and cell type on genome-editing. Sci Rep 2016; 6(1): 23549.
[http://dx.doi.org/10.1038/srep23549] [PMID: 27030102]

[21] Furugaki K, Yasuno H, Iwai T, Moriya Y, Harada N, Fujimoto-Ouchi K. Melting curve analysis for mutations of EGFR and KRAS. Anticancer Res 2014; 34(2): 613-21.
[PMID: 24510990]

[22] Duncan R, Kourout M, Grigorenko E, Fisher C, Dong M. Advances in multiplex nucleic acid diagnostics for blood-borne pathogens: promises and pitfalls. Expert Rev Mol Diagn 2016; 16(1): 83-95.
[http://dx.doi.org/10.1586/14737159.2016.1112272] [PMID: 26581018]

[23] Margulis M, Danielli A. Rapid and Sensitive Detection of Repetitive Nucleic Acid Sequences Using Magnetically Modulated Biosensors. ACS Omega 2019; 4(7): 11749-55.
[http://dx.doi.org/10.1021/acsomega.9b01071] [PMID: 31460281]

[24] Hammond JL, Bhalla N, Rafiee SD, Estrela P. Localized surface plasmon resonance as a biosensing platform for developing countries. Biosensors (Basel) 2014; 4(2): 172-88.
[http://dx.doi.org/10.3390/bios4020172] [PMID: 25587417]

[25] Zielezinski A, Vinga S, Almeida J, Karlowski WM. Alignment-free sequence comparison: benefits, applications, and tools. Genome Biol 2017; 18(1): 186.
[http://dx.doi.org/10.1186/s13059-017-1319-7] [PMID: 28974235]

[26] Shen Y, Li Y, Liu TT, Chen L. Microscopical and physicochemical identification of 3 sources of Curcumae Rhizoma. Chem Res Appl 2014; 26: 267-70.

[27] Buels R, Yao E, Diesh CM, *et al.* JBrowse: a dynamic web platform for genome visualization and analysis. Genome Biol 2016; 17(1): 66.
[http://dx.doi.org/10.1186/s13059-016-0924-1] [PMID: 27072794]

[28] Akiyoshi K, Yamada Y, Honma Y, *et al.* KRAS mutations in patients with colorectal cancer as detected by high-resolution melting analysis and direct sequencing. Anticancer Res 2013; 33(5): 2129-34.
[PMID: 23645765]

[29] Wojdacz TK. Methylation-sensitive high-resolution melting in the context of legislative requirements for validation of analytical procedures for diagnostic applications. Expert Rev Mol Diagn 2012; 12(1): 39-47.
[http://dx.doi.org/10.1586/erm.11.88] [PMID: 22133118]

[30]   Wojdacz TK, Windeløv JA, Thestrup BB, Damsgaard TE, Overgaard J, Hansen L. Identification and characterization of locus-specific methylation patterns within novel loci undergoing hypermethylation during breast cancer pathogenesis. Breast Cancer Res 2014; 16(1): R17.
[http://dx.doi.org/10.1186/bcr3612] [PMID: 24490656]

[31]   Duyvejonck H, Cools P, Decruyenaere J, *et al.* Validation of high resolution melting analysis (HRM) of the amplified ITS2 region for the detection and identification of yeasts from clinical samples: comparison with culture and MALDI-TOF based identification. PLoS One 2015; 10(8): e0132149.
[http://dx.doi.org/10.1371/journal.pone.0132149] [PMID: 26295947]

[32]   Raja HA, Miller AN, Pearce CJ, Oberlies NH. Fungal identification using molecular tools: a primer for the natural products research community. J Nat Prod 2017; 80(3): 756-70.
[http://dx.doi.org/10.1021/acs.jnatprod.6b01085] [PMID: 28199101]

[33]   Siyadat P, Ayatollahi H, Barati M, Sheikhi M, Shahidi M. High Resolution Melting Analysis for Evaluation of mir-612 (Rs12803915) Genetic Variant with Susceptibility to Pediatric Acute Lymphoblastic Leukemia. Rep Biochem Mol Biol 2021; 9(4): 385-93.
[http://dx.doi.org/10.52547/rbmb.9.4.385] [PMID: 33969131]

[34]   Prathibha VH, Hegde V, Sharadraj KM, Rajesh MK, Rachana KE, Chowdappa P. Differentiation of Phytophthora species associated with plantation crops using PCR and high-resolution melting curve analysis. J Plant Pathol 2018; 100(2).

[35]   Rojo D, Zapata M, Maureira A, Guiñez R, Wulff-Zottele C, Rivas M. High-resolution melting analysis for identification of microalgae species. J Appl Phycol 2020; 32(6): 3901-11.
[http://dx.doi.org/10.1007/s10811-020-02240-y]

[36]   Ladas I, Fitarelli-Kiehl M, Song C, *et al.* Multiplexed Elimination of Wild-Type DNA and High-Resolution Melting Prior to Targeted Resequencing of Liquid Biopsies. Clin Chem 2017; 63(10): 1605-13.
[http://dx.doi.org/10.1373/clinchem.2017.272849] [PMID: 28679646]

[37]   Liu Y. High Resolution Meltcurve PCR assay for detection of Salmonella and Escherichia coli o157: h7 in foods (Doctoral dissertation, University of Missouri--Columbia). 2017.

[38]   Pattison SH, Rogers GB, Crockard M, Elborn JS, Tunney MM. Molecular detection of CF lung pathogens: current status and future potential. J Cyst Fibros 2013; 12(3): 194-205.
[http://dx.doi.org/10.1016/j.jcf.2013.01.007] [PMID: 23402821]

[39]   Park SY, Park KH, Bang KM, *et al.* Clinical significance and outcome of polymicrobial *Staphylococcus aureus* bacteremia. J Infect 2012; 65(2): 119-27.
[http://dx.doi.org/10.1016/j.jinf.2012.02.015] [PMID: 22410381]

[40]   Pasic MD, Samaan S, Yousef GM. Genomic medicine: new frontiers and new challenges. Clin Chem 2013; 59(1): 158-67.
[http://dx.doi.org/10.1373/clinchem.2012.184622] [PMID: 23284016]

[41]   Pritchard CC, Cheng HH, Tewari M. MicroRNA profiling: approaches and considerations. Nat Rev Genet 2012; 13(5): 358-69.
[http://dx.doi.org/10.1038/nrg3198] [PMID: 22510765]

[42]   Blainey PC. The future is now: single-cell genomics of bacteria and archaea. FEMS Microbiol Rev 2013; 37(3): 407-27.
[http://dx.doi.org/10.1111/1574-6976.12015] [PMID: 23298390]

[43]   Nawar T, Kaltsas A, Tang YW. Molecular Diagnostics in Central Nervous System Infections. Neurological Complications of Infectious Diseases 2021; pp. 13-36.
[http://dx.doi.org/10.1007/978-3-030-56084-3_2]

[44]   Müller KE. Characterisation of Leishmania amino acid permease 3 (AAP3) coding sequences and flanking regions as a target of detection and diagnosis of the leishmaniases. 2020.

[45]   Fogelson SB, Camus AC, Lorenz WW, *et al*. Variation among human, veterinary and environmental Mycobacterium chelonae-abscessus complex isolates observed using core genome phylogenomic analysis, targeted gene comparison, and anti-microbial susceptibility patterns. PLoS One 2019; 14(3): e0214274.
[http://dx.doi.org/10.1371/journal.pone.0214274] [PMID: 30908517]

[46]   Sinha MB. Improving Clinical Practices in the Neonatal Intensive Care Unit: A Bioengineering Approach (Doctoral dissertation, UC San Diego).

[47]   Ozbak H, Dark P, Maddi S, Chadwick P, Warhurst G. Combined molecular gram typing and high-resolution melting analysis for rapid identification of a syndromic panel of bacteria responsible for sepsis-associated bloodstream infection. J Mol Diagn 2012; 14(2): 176-84.
[http://dx.doi.org/10.1016/j.jmoldx.2011.12.004] [PMID: 22269179]

[48]   Gago S, Zaragoza Ó, Cuesta I, Rodríguez-Tudela JL, Cuenca-Estrella M, Buitrago MJ. High-resolution melting analysis for identification of the Cryptococcus neoformans-Cryptococcus gattii complex. J Clin Microbiol 2011; 49(10): 3663-6.
[http://dx.doi.org/10.1128/JCM.01091-11] [PMID: 21832024]

[49]   Wang J, Yang J, Gao S, *et al*. Rapid detection and differentiation of Theileria annulata, T. orientalis and T. sinensis using high-resolution melting analysis. Ticks Tick Borne Dis 2020; 11(1): 101312.
[http://dx.doi.org/10.1016/j.ttbdis.2019.101312] [PMID: 31645296]

[50]   Słomka M, Sobalska-Kwapis M, Wachulec M, Bartosz G, Strapagiel D. High resolution melting (HRM) for high-throughput genotyping—limitations and caveats in practical case studies. Int J Mol Sci 2017; 18(11): 2316.
[http://dx.doi.org/10.3390/ijms18112316] [PMID: 29099791]

[51]   Lasa-Fernandez H, Mosqueira-Martín L, Alzualde A, Lasa-Elgarresta J, Vallejo-Illarramendi A. A genotyping method combining primer competition PCR with HRM analysis to identify point mutations in Duchenne animal models. Sci Rep 2020; 10(1): 17224.
[http://dx.doi.org/10.1038/s41598-020-74173-y] [PMID: 33057138]

[52]   Chakraborty S, Dutta TK, De A, Ghosh S, Das M, Banerjee A. High Resolution Melting Analysis (HRMA) and its strategic applications in Veterinary science. Indian Journal of Comparative Microbiology. Immunol Infect Dis 2019; 40(1): 1-0.

[53]   Mérida-García R, Gálvez S, Paux E, *et al*. High resolution melting and insertion site-based polymorphism markers for wheat variability analysis and candidate genes selection at drought and heat MQTL loci. Agronomy (Basel) 2020; 10(9): 1294.
[http://dx.doi.org/10.3390/agronomy10091294]

[54]   Nemcova E, Cernochova M, Ruzicka F, Malisova B, Freiberger T, Nemec P. Rapid identification of medically important Candida isolates using high resolution melting analysis. PLoS One 2015; 10(2): e0116940.
[http://dx.doi.org/10.1371/journal.pone.0116940] [PMID: 25689781]

[55]   Cousins MM, Laeyendecker O, Beauchamp G, *et al*. Use of a high resolution melting (HRM) assay to compare gag, pol, and env diversity in adults with different stages of HIV infection. PLoS One 2011; 6(11): e27211.
[http://dx.doi.org/10.1371/journal.pone.0027211] [PMID: 22073290]

[56]   James MM, Wang L, Musoke P, *et al*. Association of HIV diversity and survival in HIV-infected Ugandan infants. PLoS One 2011; 6(4): e18642.
[http://dx.doi.org/10.1371/journal.pone.0018642] [PMID: 21533179]

[57]   Chen X, Kong F, Wang Q, Li C, Zhang J, Gilbert GL. Rapid detection of isoniazid, rifampin, and ofloxacin resistance in *Mycobacterium tuberculosis* clinical isolates using high-resolution melting analysis. J Clin Microbiol 2011; 49(10): 3450-7.
[http://dx.doi.org/10.1128/JCM.01068-11] [PMID: 21832014]

[58] Kovanda A, Poljak M. Real-time polymerase chain reaction assay based on high-resolution melting analysis for the determination of the rs12979860 polymorphism involved in hepatitis C treatment response. J Virol Methods 2011; 175(1): 125-8.
[http://dx.doi.org/10.1016/j.jviromet.2011.04.018] [PMID: 21549150]

[59] Snyder SA. Emerging chemical contaminants: Looking for greater harmony. J Am Water Works Assoc 2014; 106(8): 38-52.
[http://dx.doi.org/10.5942/jawwa.2014.106.0126]

[60] Goldschmidt P, Degorge S, Che Sarria P, *et al.* New strategy for rapid diagnosis and characterization of fungal infections: the example of corneal scrapings. PLoS One 2012; 7(7): e37660.
[http://dx.doi.org/10.1371/journal.pone.0037660] [PMID: 22768289]

[61] Zhang Y, Wang Z, Li B, *et al.* High-resolution melting curve analysis for rapid detection of Isoniazid-resistant *Mycobacterium tuberculosis* in Qinghai Province. J Exp Clin Microbiol 2018.

[62] Mohammad Rahimi H, Pourhosseingholi MA, Yadegar A, Mirjalali H, Zali MR. High-resolution melt curve analysis: A real-time based multipurpose approach for diagnosis and epidemiological investigations of parasitic infections. Comp Immunol Microbiol Infect Dis 2019; 67: 101364.
[http://dx.doi.org/10.1016/j.cimid.2019.101364] [PMID: 31590033]

CHAPTER 7

Current Therapeutic Options and Challenges for MDR

Aakanksha Kalra[1], Sakshi Piplani[2] and Ravi Ranjan Kumar Niraj[3,*]

[1] *Dr B. Lal Institute of Biotechnology, Jaipur, 302017, India*

[2] *Vaxine Pty Ltd, Warradale, Australia; College of Medicine and Public Health, Flinders University, Adelaide, Australia*

[3] *Amity Institute of Biotechnology Amity University Rajasthan, Jaipur, 303002, India*

Abstract: Multiple-Drug Resistance (MDR) against many antibiotics and other therapeutic agents is a major concern for health care providers and researchers in the field. Due to tremendous rise in MDR cases, researchers are in search of potent therapeutic options or alternatives to overcome MDR. Here, in this chapter, we will discuss the current status of the common as well as advanced methods which have been developed so far for the treatment of MDR and also the challenges and opportunities in each of those methods. This chapter discusses common methods used for the treatment of MDR, *i.e.*, major antibiotics used for the treatment of MDR bacteria and synergistic approaches by the combination of different antibiotics. Along with common treatments used against MDR bacteria, this chapter also discusses current treatments like anti-microbial peptides, anti-virulence compounds, phage therapy and drug repurposing approaches for MDR treatment.

Keywords: Allopathic medicines, Anti-microbial peptide, Antibiotics, Carbapenems, Multiple-drug resistance, Phage therapy.

INTRODUCTION

The relationship between bacterial species and humans is age old, with one affecting the other in their life cycle. Many bacterial species are essential part of the human body and its metabolism; they are referred to as the normal flora. However, many more have been identified as causative agents of numerous diseases. The use of traditional medicines and antibiotics for the cure of these infections has been consistent with emerging diseases and scientific advancements. However, the identification of novel antibiotics is being rendered

---

* **Corresponding author Ravi Ranjan Kumar Niraj:** Amity Institute of Biotechnology Amity University Rajasthan, Jaipur, 303002, India; E-mail: rrkniraj@gmail.com

Sanket Kaushik and Nagendra Singh (Eds.)

ineffective with the emerging resistance to the available drugs. This antibiotic resistance is increasing at a very rapid rate, thereby classifying the resistant bacteria into three different categories, *i.e.* multidrug resistant, extreme drug resistant and pan drug resistant. Considering the severity of the situation, drug resistance is one of the major thrusts in the health sector. The focus on drug resistance globally initiated in 2011, when WHO declared "combat drug resistance: no action today, no cure tomorrow" (WHO Report 2011). This was later revised in 2015 when World Health Organization focussed on all the aspects of drug resistance, including awareness and understanding of the antimicrobial resistance in addition to its prevention and cure. Needless to say, antimicrobial resistance (AMR) has become a global health concern in the present scenario. It has affected the global progress in multiple ways, which include affecting the economically weaker sections to a great extent, causing untreatable infections even in animals in turn affecting sustainable food production and affecting healthcare systems. According to the World Bank Group Report on Drug-Resistant Infections (March 2017), the economic burden of AMR is expected to rise to about US $ 120 trillion by 2050, suggesting a dire and urgent need to focus on the issue [1]. The worldwide attempt to keep a check on the rising AMR was made in 2015 by WHO with the objective to create awareness, understanding, strengthening knowledge and evidence towards AMR; reducing the infection rates and optimizing antibiotic use of the antimicrobial agents. However, lack of funds has been the major cause of the huge difference in the national action planning vs. implementation. India is one of the countries enrolled in the Global Antimicrobial Resistance Surveillance System (GLASS) program to create awareness and keep a check on AMR. While understanding the mechanism of the emerging resistance, it has been observed that bacteria can evade the antimicrobial activity of antibiotics *via* three different but related mechanisms: resistance, tolerance and persistence. Therefore, this chapter is focussed on the current status of the traditional as well as advanced methods, which have been developed so far for the treatment of MDR and also the challenges involved in each of those methods.

TRADITIONAL METHODS USED FOR TREATMENT OF MDR

It is a well-known fact that the number of bacteria on earth greatly outnumbers the total humans and many of them are causative agents of infectious diseases. Multiple approaches have been employed since ages for the treatment of these infections. which can mostly be categorized in home remedies; *i.e.*, Ayurveda/Unani systems of medicines, homeopathy and antibiotics. The first three systems of medicines are basically focussed on the symptom derived treatment rather than focusing on the pathogen involved. On the other hand, a wide range of antibiotics has been developed since the discovery of penicillin by

Alexander Fleming in 1928, most of which have been specific to the target bacterial species. This advent of antibiotics towards bacterial species, on the one hand, had overwhelmed all the existing systems of infection treatment back then and also revolutionized the treatment process for multiple infections, but, on the other hand, its misuse and overuse have led to the emergence of drug-resistant species. The more the number of antibiotics has been discovered, the greater the emerging resistance in isolates leading to the formation of multidrug (MDR), extensive drug (XDR) and pan-drug (PDR) resistant species. The ever-rising number of such species has urged a dire need for evaluation of existing and alternative strategies to combat them. The developed antibiotics as well as the ones in the development pipeline, are discussed in great detail in next section.

The use of plant-based traditional medicines for health care can be dated to as old as 200 BCE and are responsible for meeting healthcare needs across the world. For instance, healthcare needs up to 80% of African population and 40% of Chinese population are met *via* traditional medicines (WHO report 2002). The use of herbal formulations as antibiotics is gaining attention and mixed results have been obtained for the same. Certain studies have shown these formulations to be effective [2], while others have shown these formulations to be ineffective [3]. Medicinal extracts of various plants have been evaluated against resistant species of some of the most common pathogens, such as MRSA, *Klebsiella* spp., *etc.*, and have shown promising results. Irrespective of the efficacy of the formulation, one of the most common side effects of these formulations is hepatotoxicity, which is observed due to unregulated doses of the formulations by oral route [4]. In spite of the above-mentioned concerns, the role of Ayurveda, medicinal plants and herbal formulations have been exploited as alternative strategies in the global market for a number of diseases. Together with home remedies, these alternatives have been the primary source of healthcare for a long time, but owing to their unascertained quality, lack of accurate chemical composition of the formulation, safety, efficacy, lack of regulation and unknown side effects, their use has been limited so far [3].

Major Antibiotics used for Treatment of MDR Bacteria

The discovery of antibiotics has been a long journey, and, in the process, extensive classes of antibiotics have been exploited affecting different pathways of the bacterial life cycle. The latest generation of antibiotics that are in use are discussed in this section. Depending on their mechanism of action on the bacterial life cycle, the antibiotics have been classified in the following categories:

Carbapenems

Carbapenems are a class of antibiotics belonging to beta-lactams discovered in the 1980s with the discovery of Streptomyces cattleya and its antibiotic product as thienamycin [5]. In the current scenario, these are the first line of drugs reserved towards high risk or severe bacterial infections, usually MDR ones. Similar to other antibiotics belonging to this class, they also affect the cell wall biosynthesis of the bacteria *via* binding to penicillin binding proteins (PBPs). These have been employed after the emergence of resistance to the previous generations of this antibiotic class, *viz.* penicillins and cephalosporins, at the beginning of the 21st century. Besides, they have a much broader spectrum of activity when compared to their previous generation counterparts. They have been found to be effective towards *Klebsiella, Pseudomonas* spp., *Acinetobacter* spp. and other *Enterobacteriacea* family members, which, in the present scenario, are a major cause of MDR in both the community acquired as well as hospital acquired infections as suggested by WHO Reports 2019. These are specifically effective against *Acinetobacter* spp. infections, which have shown resistance to almost all the available drugs, such as penicillin, cephalosporins, quinolones and aminoglycosides. The current members of this class in use are imipenem, meropenem and doripenem. Having said that, species resistant to carbapenems, such as carbapenem-resistant *Klebsiella pneumoniae* (CRKP), have also emerged, thereby suggesting a dire and urgent need to look out for alternatives. The mechanism of the emerging resistance towards carbapenems includes impermeability to the drug, loss of porin, and action of efflux pumps, but the production of carbapenemases is the most important one.

Polymyxins

Polymyxins are chemical peptides naturally produced by Gram-positive bacteria such as *Paenibacillus polymyxa* that are used as antibiotics, specifically towards Gram-negative bacteria such as *Pseudomonas* spp. or *Klebsiella* spp. These molecules specifically bind to the lipopolysaccharide layer of the Gram-negative bacteria, ultimately destroying both the inner as well as outer membranes of the cell, showing bactericidal effects. Since its mechanism of action is similar to that of the micelle formation by detergents, these are at times also referred to as detergents of Gram-negative bacteria. Owing to their neurotoxic as well as nephrotoxic side-effects, these are the last resort antibiotics and are used only when all other antibiotics are rendered ineffective. They are most commonly employed for carbapenem-resistant bacteria, including carbapenem-resistant Enterobacteriaceae (CRE), *Pseudomonas aeruginosa* (CRPA) and *Acinetobacter baumanii* (CRAB) [6]. Currently, the most common polymyxins include polymyxin E (colistin) and polymyxin B. Having said that, there are incidences of emerging resistance to these antibiotics as well in certain countries, which is an issue that needs to be addressed. Therefore, owing to the side-effects as well as the emerging resistance, efforts are being made to optimize the indications and the dosages of these antibiotics to increase the efficacy at the international scale.

Aminoglycosides

Aminoglycosides belong to the class of antibiotics that target protein synthesis in the bacterial cell by inhibiting the elongation step at the 30S ribosomal subunit during translation. Similar to polymyxins, these are also specifically used for Gram-negative drug-resistant bacteria. The first aminoglycoside discovered was Streptomycin which was followed by multiple similar antibiotics like gentamicin, tobramycin, neomycin, *etc.* These antibiotics work in a concentration-dependent manner and are used for carbapenem-resistant bacteria, more specifically, the ones resistant to polymyxins. The reasons behind their low usage are similar to that of polymyxins, *viz.* nephrotoxicity and reduced lung concentrations. Thus, these antibiotics also belong to the last resort drugs. Meanwhile, the emergence of resistance towards these drugs has further limited their use. However, a recent aminoglycoside, plazomicin, which is a derivative of sisomicin, has shown promising results in a number of MDR bacteria as it retains stability towards a number of aminoglycoside-modifying enzymes, the major reason for aminoglycoside resistance.

Oxazolidinone

Oxazolidinones are another category of antibiotics that affect the translation process in the bacterial cell by inhibiting the binding of N-formylmethionyl-tRNA to the ribosome. The first drug developed in this class was cycloserine which was used against tuberculosis in 1956. This was followed by the discovery of Linezolid in the 2000s, owing to the emergence of multiple drug-resistant species, especially towards the Vancomycin resistant ones. Owing to this, Linezolid was developed as the first-line drug for the treatment of VRE infections. However, the emergence of Linezolid resistant VRE in recent studies has further limited its use.

Glycylcycline

Another category of antibiotics affecting the translation process in the bacterial cells by binding to the 30S subunit of the ribosome is glycylcyclines. The first member of the class is tigecycline, developed in the early 2000s, which is a tetracycline derivative that has broader modes of action than the parent drug and thus can be used against both Gram-negative and positive bacteria. In spite of its broader spectrum towards bacteria, its usage is limited by the associated mortalities. On the basis of four randomized trials, WHO has declared a blackbox warning against the drug owing to its high mortality rate, and thus, the drug is used only in severe cases with no other antibiotics available with special care to be maintained in ventilator-associated pneumonia (VAP) [7].

Another cycline antibiotic in the developmental stage is eravacycline, a fluorocyclinesimilar to tigecycline in structure. The antibiotic is designed in a way that it is effective against a broad range of microbes, including both Gram-positive and negative ones but is ineffective towards certain bacteria such as *P. aeruginosa* and *Burkholderia cenopacia*. One of the major advantages of this drug is its efficacy towards CRAB *in vitro*, which is a global priority pathogen in the current scenario, as stated by WHO [8].

Synergistic Approach by Combination of Antibiotics

The analysis of the antibiotics developed so far and their effect on the emerging microbial species has made it very clear that alternative strategies need to be exploited to combat the bacterial catastrophes. One of the alternative strategies is using the current antibiotics in combination so as to target multiple pathways in the organisms simultaneously. In this context, multiple such combinations have been evaluated, of which some are in use while others are in exploratory phases. Some of these combinations are discussed here.

As already described previously in the chapter, carbapenems have been the first line of antibiotics in use but, owing to the emerging resistance; their use is restricted. However, some approaches have been carried out with carbapenem in combinations with other agents that have slightly higher MICs than carbapenem alone but offer efficacy towards the resistant isolates. Certain combinations of carbapenems have been shown to be efficacious towards CRE infections, particularly caused by *Klebsiella pneumonia* carbapenemase- (KPC-) producing strains but other similar trials of meropenem with colistin showed no synergy towards CRAB isolates, rendering the combination inefficacious. Owing to the limited number of such combinations tested, the ultimate conclusions cannot be made.

Another drug used in combination is fosfomycin which is a phosphoenolpyruvate analogue interfering with the peptidoglycan synthesis of the bacterial cell wall. It has been used in combination with colistin towards CRAB infections, but no significant differences were observed in the survival time [9]. Besides, owing to limited trials of the combinations as well as higher mortality rates, the drug can be reserved as the last resort for severe cases.

One of the most widely studied combinations of antibiotics is that consisting of beta lactams and beta-lactamase inhibitors (BL-BLI). Ceftazidime along with avibactam is one such combination showing activity against class A and class D carbapenemase-producing CRE and also towards CRPA isolates [10]. Owing to the positive results of the combination in the trials, it is considered an effective and important option for CRE but requires optimization as per antimicrobial stewardship principles.

Another BL-BLI combination showing efficacious results is the combination of meropenem and vaborbactam, showing promising results towards class A carbapenemase producing CRE. The combination has been approved by European Medicines Agency for complicated Urinary Tract Infections, complicated Intra-abdominal Infections, Hospital Acquired Pneumonia, VAP, and infections due to aerobic Gram-negative organisms in adult patients with limited treatment options [11]. However, the use of this combination has to be optimized, keeping in mind the rate of emerging resistance so as to ensure its use in the long run. Ceftolozane/tazobactam is yet another combination of the similar category with high potency towards CRPA *in vitro* but against the isolates producing carbapenemase or against CRE.

Aztreonam was the only available monobactam antibiotic since 1986 for Mannose Binding Lectin producing bacteria, but the antibiotic is rendered ineffective by amber class A and class C beta-lactamases *via* hydrolysis. However, its combination with avibactam has shown potent activity against Extended Spectrum β Lactamases, class C blactamase, MBL, and KPC-producing strains when compared to aztreonam alone. Owing to the limited option for MBL-producing strains, this combination, if shown efficacious, can be a promising alternative.

Bioenhancers

In addition to the exploitation of antibiotics alone, the combinations of antibiotics with other formulations or of only traditional or herbal formulations have also been evaluated [12]. In view of this, traditional medicines have been combined with modern antibiotics to offer multiple advantages. These include lesser side effects, lower cost (particularly important for developing countries), broadening of antimicrobial spectrum and prevention of drug-resistant mutant emergence. Such combinations have been referred to as bio-enhancers and they improve the efficacy *via* either of the following mechanisms:

- Increasing drug ADME (Absorption, Distribution, Metabolism, and Excretion).
- Modulating biotransformation of drugs in the liver and intestines.
- Modulating active transport phenomenon.
- Decreasing elimination.
- Boost the immune system.

CURRENT TREATMENT METHODS USED FOR TREATING PATIENTS WITH MDR BACTERIAL INFECTIONS

Use of Anti-microbial Peptides as Therapeutic Agent

Antimicrobial peptides (AMPs), also known as host defence peptides, are short in length and usually positively charged peptides found in a diversity of life forms, from microorganisms to humans. Most antimicrobial peptides have the capability to kill microbial pathogens directly, but few AMPs act indirectly by modulating the host defence systems. Due to rapidly increasing resistance development to conventional antibiotics across the world, the clinical uses of AMPs are increasing rapidly. Out of many AMPs used against MDR, only a few are discussed here as examples. Thanatin is a possible therapeutic agent against MDR pathogens. Thanatin is a 21-amino acid residue peptide and S-thanatin, an analogue of thanatin, shows potent antimicrobial activity against many strains of Gram-negative as well as Gram-positive bacteria and it also shows low hemolytic activity. Additionally, S-thanatin shows potent activity against *K. pneumoniae* and *E. coli* at minimum concentrations and can alleviate sepsis in mice models. Colistin is another important AMP used as a very promising drug for the treatment of MDR pathogen infections [13], although recently, it was reported that resistance to colistin is a concerning global health issue in the fight against MDR bacterial infections. The two newly discovered AMPs, AA139 and SET-M33, having a similar mechanism of action as colistin, have shown outstanding therapeutic potential both *in vitro* and *in vivo* experiments. Many potential AMPs with effective activity against Gram-positive and Gram-negative MDR bacteria have been isolated and characterized from marine animals. For example, mytimacin-AF, isolated from marine molluscs, shows effective activity against *S. aureus* and *K. pneumoniae*. Another one is tachyplesin, isolated from horseshoe crab hemocytes, with potent activities against MDR gram-negative and gram-positive bacteria [14 - 16].

Anti-Virulence Compounds

The resistance developed by micro-organismsagainst antimicrobial drugs produced one of the major challenges for humanity in the twenty first century.

The spread of resistant pathogens has been increased in a way that the possibility of returning to a pre-antibiotic era is true. In the current situation, novel therapeutic strategies must be developed to restrict drug resistance. Amongst the novel proposed strategies, anti-virulence therapy has been projected as a promising substitute for potent control strategies of the spread and rise of resistant pathogens. The major anti-virulence strategies include targeting quench pathogen quorum sensing (QS) systems, disassemble of bacterial functional membrane microdomains (FMMs), disruption of biofilm formation and bacterial toxin neutralization.

Some important examples of anti-virulence drug are coumarin (Anti-QS, Anti-biofilm against *P. aeruginosa* PAO1); T315 compound (Anti-biofilm against *S. enterica* serovar *Typhimurium*, *S. enterica* serovar *Typhi*, and *A. baumannii*); kaempferol (Anti-biofilm against *S. aureus*); resveratrol (Anti-toxin and Anti-QS against *S. aureus*). Anti-virulence strategies are a very promising area of research for managing MDR associated health issues globally [17].

Drug Repurposing

Drug repurposing (DR), also known as drug repositioning is a process of identifying new or more therapeutic use(s) for existing/old/available drugs. Simply, it means to find out new therapeutic uses for existing drugs. It is an effective strategy in the discovery of drug molecules with new pharmacological/therapeutic indications. It has various advantages over conventional drug discovery approaches, *i.e.*, it has reduced the reaching and development costs. It reduces the drug development timeline, as numerous existing compounds have already demonstrated safety in humans. The important thing about drug repurposing is that it does not require phase 1 clinical trials.

MDR bacteria are recognised as a global threat due to the distribution of bacteria resistant to multiple antibiotic classes. Many renowned institutions in the health sector, such as WHO and other diseases prevention and control centres have considered this situation as a global priority. Too many deaths have been recorded worldwide due to antimicrobial resistance. Data of global death due to antimicrobial resistance are available, which demand that immediate action for the development of new antimicrobial therapeutic strategies must be taken to avoid the high number of deaths predicted to occur in the future as a result of MDR bacteria. Now, it has become very important that effective solutions such as establishing antimicrobial supervising programmes, optimizing the use of existing antibiotics, discouraging the unnecessary use of antimicrobial agents, *etc.* be implemented.

Repurposing drugs have created a new interest in the treatment of certain MDR bacterial infections. It could provide a certain alternative. Repurposing drug-based approaches could be especially important for the treatment of infections caused by MDR Gram-Negative bacteria such as *Acinetobacter baumannii, Pseudomonas aeruginosa* and *Enterobacteria ceae*carbapenem-resistant for which current treatments are not active. These pathogens are classified as a critical priority for the research and development of new antibiotics [18, 19].

Phage Therapy for Treatment of MDR Bacteria

Bacteriophages are viruses that infect bacterial cells and thus have been exploited as antibacterial agents in the recent past. Having said that, it is imperative to mention here that the use of bacteriophages as antibacterial agents dates back to the 1900s, when they were in use for almost 25 years after which they were completely replaced by antibiotics [20]. However, the emerging resistance of isolates towards these antibiotics have again diverted the interest towards these phages as antibacterial agents. In spite of the fact that they have been included in the Generally Regarded As Safe (GRAS) category by the FDA in 2006, their use in humans is still limited [21]. Owing to the specificity of bacteriophages towards the bacterial cells, they amplify at the target site (specific bacteria only), affecting only the infectious phages rendering the normal flora of the body unaffected. These bacteriophages employ multiple strategies to kill the MDR bacteria. One of them is the production of endolysins that degrade the bacterial cell wall as well as biofilm formation. A purified lysin, Ply6A3, released by a novel phage, PD-6A3, effective against the resistant strains of *Acinetobacter baumanii* tested in a murine model, is one such example [22]. There are evidence which suggests that bacteriophage affects the efflux pump mechanism, thereby increasing the sensitivity of the bacteria towards traditional antibiotics [23]. This is particularly useful since efflux pump formation is one of the major resistance mechanisms employed by the majority of bacteria. Therefore, one major advantage of these phages is the targeted delivery at the infection site, thereby reducing the side effects followed by sensitizing the bacteria towards traditional drugs. Besides, other advantages of the phages include lower developmental cost, 100% bactericidal activity, lesser number of dosages required, safety, potency and specificity. Owing to the capacity for high degree of variation in the viral genome, these can also compete with the emerging resistance in the bacterial cells. Interestingly, it has also been observed that these phages have synergistic relationships with the host immune system. It is quite understood that since the life cycle of viruses depends on the viability of the bacterial cells, it never eliminates the total bacteria from the human body. However, it reduces the bacterial number to a very low extent so that the immune system is able to eliminate the total bacterial load leading to complete elimination. There are multiple examples of the effective use of bacteriophages against most common MDR bacteria, such as *Acinetobacter baumanii* or *Pseudomonas aeruginosa* [22, 24]. Apart from *A. baumanii* and *P. aeruginosa* strains, they have also shown promising results in typhoid fever and *S. Aureus* bacteremia [24]. The phages have also been entrapped within liposomes for better and efficacious results, such as those observed in *K. Pneumonia* infections [24]. The existing antibiotics have also been used in combination with phage therapy and have shown synergistic effects against MDR bacteria, suggesting the importance of synergism as well as the efficacy of each one of the processes [25].

CONCLUSION

The increasing risk of MDR is major health concern globally but many of promising new approaches like drug repurposing, anti-microbial peptides are new hope to this battel. Although, rigorous research in this field is needed to establish these new approaches as an effective weapon against MDR. The critical improvisation in traditional treatment methods of MDR and the invention and implementation of novel strategies can show cumulative impact on MDR control and treatment effort. This chapter pours a good insight into different possible approaches for the treatment of MDR. In this chapter, we discuss the current status of the traditional as well as advanced methods, which have been developed so far for the treatment of MDR. We also discussed the challenges involved in each of these methods.

CONSENT FOR PUBLICATION

Not applicable.

CONFLICT OF INTEREST

The authors declare no conflict of interest, financial or otherwise.

ACKNOWLEDGEMENTS

Declared none.

REFERENCES

[1]   Report Final, Infections Drug Resistant. A threat to our economic future 2017.

[2]   Tambekar DH, Dahikar SB. Antibacterial activity of some Indian Ayurvedic preparations against enteric bacterial pathogens. J Adv Pharm Technol Res 2011; 2(1): 24-9.
[http://dx.doi.org/10.4103/2231-4040.79801] [PMID: 22171288]

[3]   Ngemenya MN, Djeukem GGR, Nyongbela KD, *et al.* Microbial, phytochemical, toxicity analyses and

antibacterial activity against multidrug resistant bacteria of some traditional remedies sold in Buea Southwest Cameroon. BMC Complement Altern Med 2019; 19(1): 150.
[http://dx.doi.org/10.1186/s12906-019-2563-z] [PMID: 31242939]

[4]   Abdualmjid R J, Sergi C. Hepatotoxic botanicals - an evidence-based systematic review. J Pharm Pharmaceutical Sci 2013; 16(3): 376-404.
[http://dx.doi.org/10.18433/J36G6X]

[5]   Birnbaum J, Kahan FM, Kropp H, MacDonald JS. Carbapenems, a new class of beta-lactam antibiotics. Discovery and development of imipenem/cilastatin. Am J Med 1985; 78(6A): 3-21.
[http://dx.doi.org/10.1016/0002-9343(85)90097-X] [PMID: 3859213]

[6]   Bassetti M, Peghin M, Vena A, Giacobbe DR. Treatment of Infections Due to MDR Gram-Negative Bacteria. Front Med (Lausanne) 2019; 6: 74.
[http://dx.doi.org/10.3389/fmed.2019.00074] [PMID: 31041313]

[7]   Dixit D, Madduri RP, Sharma R. The role of tigecycline in the treatment of infections in light of the new black box warning. Expert Rev Anti Infect Ther 2014; 12(4): 397-400.
[http://dx.doi.org/10.1586/14787210.2014.894882] [PMID: 24597542]

[8]   Ozger HS, Cuhadar T, Yildiz SS, *et al.* In vitro activity of eravacycline in combination with colistin against carbapenem-resistant A. baumannii isolates. J Antibiot (Tokyo) 2019; 72(8): 600-4.
[http://dx.doi.org/10.1038/s41429-019-0188-6] [PMID: 31028352]

[9]   Sirijatuphat R, Thamlikitkul V. Preliminary study of colistin versus colistin plus fosfomycin for treatment of carbapenem-resistant Acinetobacter baumannii infections. Antimicrob Agents Chemother 2014; 58(9): 5598-601.
[http://dx.doi.org/10.1128/AAC.02435-13] [PMID: 24982065]

[10]   Montravers P, Bassetti M. The ideal patient profile for new beta-lactam/beta-lactamase inhibitors. Curr Opin Infect Dis 2018; 31(6): 587-93.
[http://dx.doi.org/10.1097/QCO.0000000000000490] [PMID: 30299359]

[11]   Papp-Wallace KM. The latest advances in β-lactam/β-lactamase inhibitor combinations for the treatment of Gram-negative bacterial infections. Expert Opin Pharmacother 2019; 20(17): 2169-84.
[http://dx.doi.org/10.1080/14656566.2019.1660772] [PMID: 31500471]

[12]   Appendino G, Minassi A, Taglialatela-Scafati O. Recreational drug discovery: natural products as lead structures for the synthesis of smart drugs. Nat Prod Rep 2014; 31(7): 880-904.
[http://dx.doi.org/10.1039/c4np00010b] [PMID: 24823967]

[13]   MacNair CR, Stokes JM, Carfrae LA, *et al.* Overcoming mcr-1 mediated colistin resistance with colistin in combination with other antibiotics. Nat Commun 2018; 9(1): 458.
[http://dx.doi.org/10.1038/s41467-018-02875-z] [PMID: 29386620]

[14]   Mahlapuu M, Björn C, Ekblom J. Antimicrobial peptides as therapeutic agents: opportunities and challenges. Crit Rev Biotechnol 2020; 40(7): 978-92.
[http://dx.doi.org/10.1080/07388551.2020.1796576] [PMID. 32781848]

[15]   Mahlapuu M, Håkansson J, Ringstad L, Björn C. Antimicrobial Peptides: An Emerging Category of Therapeutic Agents. Front Cell Infect Microbiol 2016; 6: 194.
[http://dx.doi.org/10.3389/fcimb.2016.00194] [PMID: 28083516]

[16]   Mwangi J, Hao X, Lai R, Zhang ZY. Antimicrobial peptides: new hope in the war against multidrug resistance. Zool Res 2019; 40(6): 488-505.
[http://dx.doi.org/10.24272/j.issn.2095-8137.2019.062] [PMID: 31592585]

[17]   Fleitas Martínez O, Cardoso MH, Ribeiro SM, Franco OL. Recent advances in anti-virulence therapeutic strategies with a focus on dismantling bacterial membrane microdomains, toxin neutralization, quorum-sensing interference and Biofilm Inhibition. Front Cell Infect Microbiol 2019; 9: 74.
[http://dx.doi.org/10.3389/fcimb.2019.00074] [PMID: 31001485]

[18] Rudrapal M, Khairnar SJ, Jadhav AG. Drug repurposing (DR): An emerging approach in drug discovery, drug repurposing - hypothesis, molecular aspects and therapeutic applications. IntechOpen 2020.https://www.intechopen.com/chapters/72744
[http://dx.doi.org/10.5772/intechopen.93193]

[19] Andrea Vila Domínguez, Manuel Enrique Jiménez Mejías, Younes Smani. Drugs Repurposing for Multi-Drug Resistant Bacterial Infections, Drug Repurposing - Hypothesis, Molecular Aspects and Therapeutic Applications, Farid A. Badria. IntechOpen 2020. https://www.intechopen.com/chapters/73248
[http://dx.doi.org/10.5772/intechopen.93635]

[20] Lin DM, Koskella B, Lin HC. Phage therapy: An alternative to antibiotics in the age of multi-drug resistance. World J Gastrointest Pharmacol Ther 2017; 8(3): 162-73.
[http://dx.doi.org/10.4292/wjgpt.v8.i3.162] [PMID: 28828194]

[21] Wang J, Hu B, Xu M, *et al.* Therapeutic effectiveness of bacteriophages in the rescue of mice with extended spectrum β-lactamase-producing *Escherichia coli* bacteremia. Int J Mol Med 2006; 17(2): 347-55.
[http://dx.doi.org/10.3892/ijmm.17.2.347] [PMID: 16391836]

[22] Wu M, Hu K, Xie Y, *et al.* A novel phage PD-6A3, and its endolysin Ply6A3, with extended lytic activity against Acinetobacter baumannii. Front Microbiol 2019; 9: 3302.
[http://dx.doi.org/10.3389/fmicb.2018.03302] [PMID: 30687281]

[23] Chan BK, Sistrom M, Wertz JE, Kortright KE, Narayan D, Turner PE. Phage selection restores antibiotic sensitivity in MDR *Pseudomonas aeruginosa*. Sci Rep 2016; 6(1): 26717.
[http://dx.doi.org/10.1038/srep26717] [PMID: 27225966]

[24] Vivas R, Barbosa AAT, Dolabela SS, Jain S. Multidrug-resistant bacteria and alternative methods to control them: An overview. Microb Drug Resist 2019; 25(6): 890-908.
[http://dx.doi.org/10.1089/mdr.2018.0319] [PMID: 30811275]

[25] Kirienko NV, Rahme L, Cho YH. Editorial: Beyond antimicrobials: Non-traditional approaches to combating multidrug-resistant bacteria. Front Cell Infect Microbiol 2019; 9: 343.
[http://dx.doi.org/10.3389/fcimb.2019.00343] [PMID: 31681623]

CHAPTER 8

Phytomedicines for Bacterial Infections

Vijay Pal¹, Ravneet Chug¹, Kumar Sambhav Verma¹, Priyal Sharma¹ and **Vinod Singh Gour¹,***

¹ Amity Institute of Biotechnology, Amity University Rajasthan, NH 11 C Kant Kalwar, Jaipur, India

Abstract: Microbial pathogens have always been a great threat to many life forms, including human. To control microbial infection, especially bacterial infection antibiotics have been a boon. However, with the changing scenario, the bacteria have also evolved and developed resistance against many antibiotics and these pathogens have become more fatal. On the other hand, plants and plant products have been used as a natural resource to control these microbes. The plant seed oil has also been explored for the same; however, comparatively less literature is available on antimicrobial activities of seed oil derived from plants. Looking at the importance of seed oil in this field, the present review article presents a brief discussion about various aspects of seed oil and their application against bacteria.

Keywords: Multidrug resistance, Phytochemicals, Plants oil, Secondary metabolites, Traditional methods.

INTRODUCTION

The discovery of a wide range of antibiotics has been considered one of the biggest accomplishments in the field of medicine. These are pivotal for treating various bacterial infections in patients, including those undergoing surgery, in intensive care units, undergoing organ grafting or in cancer treatment [1, 2]. Antibiotics are generally target specific as they affect cell wall synthesis, DNA replication, and translational machinery of the bacterial cell. Alternatively, bacteria have also developed resistance mechanisms due to the increasing human population, overuse of antimicrobials, over prescription by clinicians, public perception, and behaviour (Non-prescription purchase, not completing the antibiotic dosage as prescribed by clinicians) and commercial pressure [3]. The development of antimicrobial resistance (AMR), which is a matter of grave concern as it results in the huge loss to individuals and economy [3, 4]. Antimicrobial resistance (AMR) has been identified by the World Health Organis-

---

* **Corresponding author Vinod Singh Gour:** Amity Institute of Biotechnology, Amity University Rajasthan, NH 11 C Kant Kalwar, Jaipur India; E-mail: vkgaur@jpr.amity.edu

Sanket Kaushik and Nagendra Singh (Eds.)

ation as a global threat because ~30,000 women and ~400,000 new-born babies lose their lives due to bacterial infection (WHO, 2016). According to the AR Threats (Report-2019 of CDC) antibiotic-resistant microorganisms can lead to > 2.8 million infections and 35,000 deaths in the United States each year [5]. Antibiotic resistance also increases the challenge of recalcitrant infections.

In today's era, the rapid emergence of multidrug resistance (MDR) in microorganisms is an increasing global crisis as it poses a challenge to the treatment of infectious diseases [2, 6]. This alarming situation has enforced the scientists and medical professionals to shift from broad-spectrum empirical therapy (use of known antibiotics), which are less effective against MDR bacteria, to the personalized and strategic approach [4]. Natural compounds have always been relied upon and widely searched for the novel drug discoveries for more than 5,000 years. Plants have been extensively used as a source of antibiotics, antineoplastic, analgesics, and cardioprotective. About 70–90% of the human population in developing countries still use medicines derived from plant extracts [3, 7, 8].

In the last two decades, many persistent efforts have been made to discover novel therapeutics for combating MDR. Natural products and their derivatives contribute to more than half of the Food and Drug Administration (FDA) approved drugs [3, 9]. A variety of plants extracts have antimicrobial properties [10]. These may be bactericidal as well as bacteriostatic against microbial flux pump, quorum sensing and bio-film formation [10].

Diterpenes, extracted from root bark of *Berberis aristata* were found to have antimicrobial properties against several bacterial strains including *Enterococcus faecalis, Staphylococcus spp., Escherichia coli, Klebsiella spp., Pseudomonas aeruginosa, Salmonella spp., Shigella fexneri* at a low concentration (0.05–5 mg/mL) at the same time these diterpenes had IC_{50} value of 245 to 473 µg/mL against L20B, RD and Hep 2 cell lines, indicating higher biosafety level [11]. Similar to this Arora and Sood (2017) [12] reported the leaf extracts of *Gymnema sylvester* to have antimicrobial activities against *Klebsiella pneumoniae* and *Staphylococcus epidermidis*, further they reported the safety of these extracts based on MTT assay and Ame's test. So, it can be stated that the herbal drugs are more efficient and less toxic to various cell lines; hence, they may be explored to replace the less effective antibiotics and/or antibiotics with threatening side effects. Therefore, herbal compounds provide a novel and promising alternative source of antibiotics against microbial agents. The current review highlights the antibacterial activity of the various seed oil extracted from plants against different bacteria.

TREES AND SEED OIL

Plants mainly propagate through seeds. The seeds may contain nucellus and/or endosperm along with embryo. The nucellar and endosperm tissue contains good amount of stored nutrients, which facilitates the germination of the seed and development of the seedling till the development of first leaf. This reserve food includes carbohydrates, proteins, and lipids. Some tree seeds are rich in oil content.

The lipids are high energy molecules stored by the plants. In perennial trees, the seed oil has been reported from many plants like *Balanites aegyptiaca*, *Azadirachta indica*, *Jatropha curcas*, *Citrus spp.*, and *Paeonia spp* [13 - 17]. The amount of the oil in seeds may vary from 13.74% to 54.37% in plants like *Jatropha curcas* and *Paeonia ostia* [15, 17]. The oil mainly consist of fatty acids, but it also possesses a small quantity of secondary metabolites, which may serve as nutraceuticals and/or drugs to treat various diseases, including bacterial infections.

SEED OIL CHEMICAL COMPOSITION

Neem seed oil contains the following fatty acids: linoleic acid (34.69%), oleic acid (20.46%), stearic acid (20.42%), palmitic acid (18.66%), arachidic acid (3.59%) behenic acid (0.80%), lignoceric acid (0.55%) and palmitic-oleic acid 0.17% [18]. According to Cesa *et al.* (2019), high pressure liquid chromatography-based chemical analysis of the pure neem oil revealed that it had no phenolic acids [19]. Neem oil had ~24 µg/mL polyphenols, where benzoic acid (12.6µg/mL) and t-cinnamic acid (1.9µg/mL) were found to be the most abundant.

Ahmed *et al.* (2008) studied seed oil composition based on gas chromatography/ mass spectrometry (GC/MS) in *Salvadora persica* collected from Gabal Elba, a mountain in East South Egypt [20]. They found that the oil contains mainly heptadecene-8-carbonic acid (~39%), indole (18%), hexadecanoic acid (13%) and octadecanoic acid (8%). Table **1** depicts the detail of seed oils obtained from some trees and their composition.

Table 1. Seed oil, fatty acid composition and other active principles.

S.No	Plant	Oil (%)	Fatty Acid Composition	Active Principles	References
01	*Calophyllum inophyllum*	33.46%-58.19%	Monoglycerol, sn-1-3 diacyleglyceroles, sn1-2 diacylglyceroles,tryglyceroles, steroles	Crude oil, Acetonide, Methanolic and n- Hexane extract	[21]
02	*Azadirachta indica*		Linealicacid, oleicacid, stearic, palmitic, arachidic,behenic,lignoceric, palmeatelic acid	Azadirachitin, nimbin, salanin	[22]
03	*Murraya koenigi*	85.4%	Oleic acid, linoleic acid, palmiticacid, stearic acid.	Carbozole and crude oil. carbazole alkaloids, kurryam (**I**), koenimbine (**II**) and koenine (**III**).	[23]
04	*Prosopis cineraria*	10.6%	Saturated fatty acid, unsaturated fatty acid, methyl hydroxyl fatty, linoleic acid, oleic acid	Crude oil.	[24]
05	*Prosopis juliflora*	7.8%	Palmitic acid, stearic acid, oleic acid, linolenic acid	Crude oil	[25]
06	*Tecomella undulata*	7.14%(44.5% fatty acid)	Linoleic acid, oleic acid, stearic acid, palmitic acid	Crude oil	[26]
07	*Salvadora persica*	40%	Lauric acid, myristic acid, palmitic acid, oleicacid		[27]
08	*Capparis decidua*	20%	Palmitic, palmitoleic, stearic, oleic, linoleic,linolenic	Tocopheroles, glucosinolate oilic, vaccinic acid with vitamin c	[28]
09	*Moringa olifera*	35%- 45%	Oleic acid, polyunsaturated fatty acid caprylic,myristic,palmitic,palmitoleic, margaric, stearic,oleic acid,linolenic, linoleic acid,arachidic,gadoleic,behenic, erucic,lignoceric,cerotic	Methanolic extract, moringine	[29]
10	*Ailanthus excelsa*		Myristic acid, palmitic palmitolic, stearic, oleic, linoleic, linolenic, arachidic, eicosenic	Crude oil	[30]
11	*Balanites aegyptiaca*	45- 46%	Palmitic acid, stearic, oleic acid, linoleic acid	Crude oil	[31]

ANTIMICROBIAL ACTIVITIES IN SEED OIL

According to Sandanasamy *et al*. (2013), when bacteria were exposed to neem oil (100 mg/ml), it created a zone of inhibition of 11.7 mm for *Escherichia coli* and 13.0 mm for *Staphylococcus aureus* [18]. When *Carnobacterium maltaromaticum, Brochothrix thermosphacta, Escherichia coli, Pseudomonas fluorescens, Lactobacillus curvatus* and *Lactobacillus sakei* were exposed to a volume of 10 µl of neem oil in 100 µl liquid medium, it resulted in minimum ~89% growth reduction in each case with reference to control where neem oil was not used [32]. Based on these results, they advocated the utilization of neem oil in preservation of meat. The effect of neem oil on 48 enteropathogenic *E. coli* isolates was studied, and it was found that as the neem oil amount is increased from 0.1 µl, 1.0 µl, 10 µl and 100 µl, the percentage of bacterial growth get reduced [33]. They also reported that the zone of inhibition ranged from ~10 mm to ~30 mm when the disc is loaded with 100 µl of neem oil [27]. The neem oil had no activity against *Helicobacter pylori* [13].

Khoobchandani *et al*. (2010) demonstrated that *Eruca sativa* seed oil has most promising antimicrobial activities in comparison to other plant part extracts [34]. *E. sativa* seed oil had antimicrobial activity against antibiotic resistant Gram-negative (*Shigella flexneri, Escherichia coli and Pseudomoms aeruginosa*) and Gram-positive (*Bacillus subtilis* and *Staphylococcus aureus*) bacteria. Seed oil displayed the maximum inhibition of 74–97% for Gram-negative bacteria and 97% for Gram-positive bacteria with reference to standard antibiotic (ciprofloxacin) used. Minimum inhibitory concentration of seed oil was 60–70 µg/ml and 65-70 µg/ml for Gram-positive and Gram-negative bacteria, respectively. Antimicrobial activity of seed oil obtained from trees has been listed in Table **2**.

Table 2. Seed oil and antibacterial activities.

S. No	Plant	Bacteria	Activity	Remarks	References
01	*Callophyllum inophyllum*	*E. coli, S. typhi, P. aeruginosa, S. aureus.*	Inhibit the growth of bacteria	Death of Gram positive bacteria by protoplast leakage and Gram negative by increase release of β defensin by macrophages	[35]
02	*Pterocarpus osun*	*S. aureus*, P. aeruginosa, Mycobacterium smegmatis, S. typhi.	Inhibit the growth of bacteria	Shows the line of inhibition by disc diffusion method	[35]

(Table 2) cont.....

S. No	Plant	Bacteria	Activity	Remarks	References
03	*Prosopis cineria, P. julifora, P. grandulosa*	*E. coli, K. pneumonic, S. aureus*	Growth inhibition	Mechanism not mentioned	[25]
04	*Moringa oleifera*	*S. aureus*, B. substilis, P. aeruginosa, E. coli	Growth inhibition	Methanolic extract cause death of bacteria	[36]
05	*Capparis sps*	*Vibrio cholera, Vibrio ogava,* And multidrug resitance *E. coli*	Antibacterial activity	Mechanism not mentioned	[28]
06	*Balanites aegyptiaca*	Gram positive and Gram negative bacteria Herpes virus	Antibacterial activity, Growth inhibitor for virus	Balanintine an active compound shows anticancerous properties	[25]
07	*Murraya koenghii*	Antibacterial	Growth inhibitor	Carbazole alkaloids, kurryam (**I**), koenimbine (**II**) and koenine (**III**).	[37]

E. sativa seed oil has great pharmacological value which is due to the presence of bio-active components [34]. Seed oil of *E. sativa* consist of bio-active isothiocyanates and pertinent amount of free erucic acid [34]. The antimicrobial potential of seed oil ensures its use in the traditional medicine. It can be used for the treatment of fever, diarrhoea, urinary infection and skin infection [34].

Similarly, Alqahtani *et al.* (2019) also studied the seed oil of *Lepidium Sativum* and demonstrated antimicrobial activities [38]. To test the antimicrobial activity, microdilution method was used against *Bacillus subtilis, Klebsiella pneumoniae, Staphylococcus aureus*, Escherichia coli, Salmonella enterica, Candida albicans and *Pseudomonas aeruginosa*. Chemical analysis showed that the main constituents of the seed oil were 7,10,13- hexadecatrienoic acid, behenic acid, 11-octadecenoic acid and 7,10-hexadecadienoic acid. The minimum inhibitory concentration (MIC) for *Salmonella enterica* was 90 mg/ml and, for the rest of the pathogens, it was 47.5 mg/ml. The result of the study revealed that the seed oil could be an important source of bioactive compounds. To develop the complementary phytochemical strategies, there is an urgent need to examine the herbs for their antimicrobial activity. Derivatives of seed oils obtained from trees have also been used as antimicrobial agents and they are listed in Table **3**.

Table 3. Seed oil derivatives and antibacterial activities.

S. No	Plant	Bacteria	Derivative	Amount of Derivative	References
01	*Azadirachata indica*	*E. coli, S. aureus*	Azadirachtin, nimbin, salanin, Tetranortiri terpenoid shows antifungal activity		[22]
02	*Murraya koenigi*	Gram positive bacteria	Carbozole	--	[23]
03	*Capparis sps*	*Vibrio sps,* multidrug resistance *E. coli*	Tocopherole glucosinolate & vaccinic acid with vitamin c	aglycone of which shows high antibacterial activity (25 µg/ml)	[22]
04	*Balanites aegyptiaca*	Gram positive and negative bacteria	Balaninte and saponine		[31]

CONCLUSION AND FUTURE PROSPECTS

Due to the presence of natural medicinal chemicals in the seed oil of the plants and herbal extracts, they have important role in modern medicine, even as antimicrobial agents. In total, 80% of the world population uses traditional medicines, especially herbs, for primary healthcare.

The seed oil obtained from certain plants is rich in fatty acids. The composition of fatty acid involves saturated, unsaturated and monounsaturated fatty acids. Along with these fatty acids, the presence of many non-polar substances has been recorded in seed oil of many plants. The fatty acids, their derivatives and other active compounds have been explored for therapeutic purposes, especially against microbes, including fungi and bacteria. Further research in this field will facilitate discoveries of new molecules to control bacterial infections.

CONSENT FOR PUBLICATION

Not applicable.

CONFLICT OF INTEREST

The authors declare no conflict of interest, financial or otherwise.

ACKNOWLEDGEMENTS

Declared none.

REFERENCES

[1]   Singh A, Gautam PK, Verma A, *et al*. Green synthesis of metallic nanoparticles as effective alternatives to treat antibiotics resistant bacterial infections: A review. Biotechnol Rep (Amst) 2020; 25: e00427.
[http://dx.doi.org/10.1016/j.btre.2020.e00427] [PMID: 32055457]

[2]   Makabenta JMV, Nabawy A, Li CH, Schmidt-Malan S, Patel R, Rotello VM. Nanomaterial-based therapeutics for antibiotic-resistant bacterial infections. Nat Rev Microbiol 2021; 19(1): 23-36.
[http://dx.doi.org/10.1038/s41579-020-0420-1] [PMID: 32814862]

[3]   Anand U, Jacobo-Herrera N, Altemimi A, Lakhssassi N. A comprehensive review on medicinal plants as antimicrobial therapeutics: potential avenues of biocompatible drug discovery. Metabolites 2019; 9(11): 258.
[http://dx.doi.org/10.3390/metabo9110258] [PMID: 31683833]

[4]   Brown ED, Wright GD. Antibacterial drug discovery in the resistance era. Nature 2016; 529(7586): 336-43.
[http://dx.doi.org/10.1038/nature17042] [PMID: 26791724]

[5]   Antibiotic Resistance Threats in the United States. Atlanta, GA: U.S. Department of Health and Human Services, CDC 2019.
[http://dx.doi.org/10.15620/cdc:82532]

[6]   Michael CA, Dominey-Howes D, Labbate M. The antimicrobial resistance crisis: causes, consequences, and management. Front Public Health 2014; 2: 145.
[http://dx.doi.org/10.3389/fpubh.2014.00145] [PMID: 25279369]

[7]   Chin YW, Balunas MJ, Chai HB, Kinghorn AD. Drug discovery from natural sources. AAPS J 2006; 8(2): E239-53.
[http://dx.doi.org/10.1007/BF02854894] [PMID: 16796374]

[8]   Newman DJ, Cragg GM. Natural products as sources of new drugs from 1981 to 2014. J Nat Prod 2016; 79(3): 629-61.
[http://dx.doi.org/10.1021/acs.jnatprod.5b01055] [PMID: 26852623]

[9]   Chavan SS, Damale MG, Devanand B. Antibacterial and antifungal drugs from natural source: A review of clinical development. Natural Products in Clinical Trials: Sharjah, UAE 2018; 1: 114.
[http://dx.doi.org/10.2174/9781681082134118010006]

[10]   Savoia D. Plant-derived antimicrobial compounds: alternatives to antibiotics. Future Microbiol 2012; 7(8): 979-90.
[http://dx.doi.org/10.2217/fmb.12.68] [PMID: 22913356]

[11]   Sood H, Kumar Y, Gupta VK, Arora DS. Scientific validation of the antimicrobial and antiproliferative potential of *Berberis aristata* DC root bark, its phytoconstituents and their biosafety. AMB Express 2019; 9(1): 143.
[http://dx.doi.org/10.1186/s13568-019-0868-4] [PMID: 31512002]

[12]   Arora DS, Sood H. In vitro antimicrobial potential of extracts and phytoconstituents from *Gymnema sylvestre* R.Br. leaves and their biosafety evaluation. AMB Express 2017; 7(1): 115.
[http://dx.doi.org/10.1186/s13568-017-0416-z] [PMID: 28587443]

[13]   Habieballa AG, Alebead HE, Koko MK, Ibrahim AS, Wady AF. Antimicrobial activity and physicochemical properties of *Balanites aegyptiaca* seed oil. Eur J Chem 2021; 12(4): 450-3.
[http://dx.doi.org/10.5155/eurjchem.12.4.450-453.2142]

[14]   Elizabeth Babatunde D, Otusemade GO, Elizabeth Ojewumi M, Agboola O, Oyeniyi E, Deborah Akinlabu K. Antimicrobial activity and phytochemical screening of neem leaves and lemon grass essential oil extracts. Int J Mech Eng Tech 2019; 10(3).

[15]   Rachana S, Tarun A, Rinki R, Neha A, Meghna R. Comparative analysis of antibacterial activity of Jatropha curcas fruit parts. J Pharma Biomed Sci 2012; 15(15): 1-4.

[16]   Ndayishimiye J, Lim DJ, Chun BS. Antioxidant and antimicrobial activity of oils obtained from a mixture of citrus by-products using a modified supercritical carbon dioxide. J Ind Eng Chem 2018; 57: 339-48.
[http://dx.doi.org/10.1016/j.jiec.2017.08.041]

[17]   Zhou JX, Braun MS, Wetterauer P, Wetterauer B, Wink M. Antioxidant, cytotoxic, and antimicrobial activities of *Glycyrrhiza glabra* L., *Paeonia lactiflora* Pall., and *Eriobotrya japonica* (Thunb.) Lindl. extracts. Medicines (Basel) 2019; 6(2): 43.
[http://dx.doi.org/10.3390/medicines6020043] [PMID: 30935079]

[18]   Sandanasamy JD, Nour AH, Tajuddin SN, Hamid Nour A. Fatty acid composition and antibacterial activity of neem (Azadirachta indica) seed oil. The Open Conference Proceedings Journal. 2013; 4: pp. (1)43-8.

[19]   Cesa S, Sisto F, Zengin G, *et al.* Phytochemical analyses and pharmacological screening of Neem oil. S Afr J Bot 2019; 120: 331-7.
[http://dx.doi.org/10.1016/j.sajb.2018.10.019]

[20]   Ahmed SS, El-Gengaihi SE, Ibrahim ME, Schnug E. Preliminary phytochemical and propagation trial with Salvadora persica L. Landbauforsch Völkenrode 2008; 58(1/2): 135.

[21]   Balogun AM, Fetuga BL. Fatty acid composition of seed oils of some members of the Leguminosae family. Food Chem 1985; 17(3): 175-82.
[http://dx.doi.org/10.1016/0308-8146(85)90066-4]

[22]   Baswa M, Rath CC, Dash SK, Mishra RK. Antibacterial activity of Karanj (*Pongamia pinnata*) and Neem (*Azadirachta indica*) seed oil: a preliminary report. Microbios 2001; 105(412): 183-9.
[PMID: 11414503]

[23]   Gahlawat DK, Jakhar S, Dahiya P. Murraya koenigii (L.) Spreng: An ethnobotanical, phytochemical and pharmacological review. J Pharmacogn Phytochem 2014; 3(3): 109-19.

[24]   Gangal S, Sharma S, Rauf A. Fatty acid composition of *Prosopis cineraria* seeds. Chem Nat Compd 2009; 45(5): 705-7.
[http://dx.doi.org/10.1007/s10600-009-9425-8]

[25]   Imam R, Rafiq M, Sheng Z, *et al.* Evaluation of Physicochemical Properties and Antimicrobial Activity of Essential Oils from Seeds of *Prosopis juliflora, P. glandulosa* and *P. cineraria.* J Essent Oil-Bear Plants 2019; 22(2): 554-62.
[http://dx.doi.org/10.1080/0972060X.2019.1618203]

[26]   Kumawat R, Sharma S, Kumar S. An overview for various aspects of multifaceted, health care *Tecomella undulata* Seem. plant. Acta Pol Pharm 2012; 69(5): 993-6.
[PMID: 23061298]

[27]   Ramadan K, Alshamrani S. Phytochemical analysis and antioxidant activity of *Salvadora persica* extracts. Journal of Basic and Applied Research in Biomedicine 2016; 2(3): 390-5.

[28]   Singh P, Mishra G, Srivastava S, Jha KK, Khosa RL. Traditional uses, phytochemistry and pharmacological properties of *Capparis decidua*: An overview. Pharm Lett 2011; 3(2): 71-82.

[29]   Leone A, Spada A, Battezzati A, Schiraldi A, Aristil J, Bertoli S. Moringa oleifera seeds and oil: Characteristics and uses for human health. Int J Mol Sci 2016; 17(12): 2141.
[http://dx.doi.org/10.3390/ijms17122141] [PMID: 27999405]

[30]   Anjaneyulu B, Kaki SS, Kanjilal S, *et al.* Physico-chemical characterization and biodiesel preparation from seed oil. Energy Sources A Recovery Util Environ Effects 2017; 39(8): 811-6.
[http://dx.doi.org/10.1080/15567036.2016.1266419]

[31]   Chothani DL, Vaghasiya HU. A review on *Balanites aegyptiaca* Del (desert date): phytochemical constituents, traditional uses, and pharmacological activity. Pharmacogn Rev 2011; 5(9): 55-62.
[http://dx.doi.org/10.4103/0973-7847.79100] [PMID: 22096319]

[32]   Del Serrone P, Toniolo C, Nicoletti M. (A) Neem (*Azadirachta indica A. Juss*) Oil: A natural preservative to control meat spoilage. Foods 2015; 4(1): 3-14.
[http://dx.doi.org/10.3390/foods4010003] [PMID: 28231186]

[33]   Del Serrone P, Toniolo C, Nicoletti M. Neem (*Azadirachta indica A. Juss*) oil to tackle enteropathogenic *Escherichia coli*. BioMed Res Int 2015; 2015: 343610.
[http://dx.doi.org/10.1155/2015/343610] [PMID: 26064900]

[34]   Khoobchandani M, Ojeswi BK, Ganesh N, *et al.* Antimicrobial properties and analytical profile of traditional Eruca sativa seed oil: Comparison with various aerial and root plant extracts. Food Chem 2010; 120(1): 217-24.
[http://dx.doi.org/10.1016/j.foodchem.2009.10.011]

[35]   Adewuyi A, Fasusi OH, Oderinde RA. Antibacterial activities of acetonides prepared from the seed oils of *Calophyllum inophyllum* and *Pterocarpus osun*. Journal of Acute Medicine 2014; 4(2): 75-80.
[http://dx.doi.org/10.1016/j.jacme.2014.02.001]

[36]   Saadabi AM, Zaid IA. An in vitro antimicrobial activity of *Moringa oleifera* L. seed extracts against different groups of microorganisms. Aust J Basic Appl Sci 2011; 5(5): 129-34.

[37]   Mandal S, Nayak A, Kar M, *et al.* Antidiarrhoeal activity of carbazole alkaloids from *Murraya koenigii Spreng* (Rutaceae) seeds. Fitoterapia 2010; 81(1): 72-4.
[http://dx.doi.org/10.1016/j.fitote.2009.08.016] [PMID: 19695314]

[38]   Alqahtani FY, Aleanizy FS, Mahmoud AZ, *et al.* Chemical composition and antimicrobial, antioxidant, and anti-inflammatory activities of *Lepidium sativum* seed oil. Saudi J Biol Sci 2019; 26(5): 1089-92.
[http://dx.doi.org/10.1016/j.sjbs.2018.05.007] [PMID: 31303845]

CHAPTER 9

Molecular Mechanisms of Antimicrobial Resistance and New Targets to Address Current Drug Resistance

Divyapriya Karthikeyan[1], Sudhir Kumar Pal[1], Mukesh Kumar[2], Kali Kishore Reddy Tetala[1], Punit Kaur[2] and Sanjit Kumar[1,*]

[1] Centre for Bio Separation Technology (CBST), Vellore Institute of Technology, Vellore, Tamil Nadu, India

[2] Department of Biophysics, All India Institute of Medical Sciences, New Delhi, India

Abstract: Penicillin discovery has put forward great expectations and hope for the treatment of several infectious diseases. Inappropriate and excess use of antibiotics has led to the emergence of antibiotic-resistant (AMR) worldwide, which has become one of the greatest threats to global health. However, in the late 1940s, after approval, mass production (lead to reduced cost) and supply (lead to easy access to all people) led to the emergence of Antimicrobial Resistance (AMR). A similar behavioral pattern ensued as other classes of antibiotics were discovered (through increasing utilization to resistance). Substandard infection control practices in public healthcare settings eased the spread and transmission of resistant organisms and intensified antimicrobials' effect. The healthcare community responded with two major programs – Infection Control in the 1980s and Antimicrobial Stewardship (in the last decade). These programs depend on the end-user; however, while the importance of such global control and prevention programs cannot be disputed, these efforts alone are insufficient against the advent of AMR. Also, drug discovery has suffered from a shortage of exploitable bacterial target sites, leading to the slow evolution of novel potent drugs.

Keywords: Antibiotics, Antimicrobials, Antimicrobial resistance, Colistin-resistant, ESKAPE organism, Pan-resistant bacteria, Superbugs.

INTRODUCTION

A pathogen or an infectious agent is a biological agent that can be catastrophic and sometimes lethal to the host (both unicellular and multicellular organisms). These infectious diseases are caused by varied living agents (pathogens), which can be categorized into 5 groups namely bacteria, viruses, protozoa, fungi, and

---

* **Corresponding author Sanjit Kumar:** Centre for Bio Separation Technology (CBST), Vellore Institute of Technology, Vellore, Tamil Nadu, India; E-mail: sanjitkrroy@gmail.com

Sanket Kaushik and Nagendra Singh (Eds.)

helminths (worms). Protozoa and worms are usually associated as parasites, whereas bacteria, viruses, and fungi are collectively known as microbes. They can grow in diverse body sections, out of which the major two can be delineated as intracellular and extracellular [1].

To subdue the effects caused by these pathogens (micro-organisms), drugs such as antimicrobials are prescribed. Antimicrobials are the broad classes of substances (natural, semi-synthetic, and synthetic) that act against microorganisms. As a part of antimicrobials, there is also another class of drugs called antibiotics [2], which attributes to the materials generated only by the microbes that work in contradictor to another microbe [3]. Antimicrobials comprise antibiotics, antivirals, antifungals, and antiparasitics. These agents have been in use for so many years to treat infections and wounds [4]. The introduction of these agents, such as sulphonamides (1935), penicillin (in 1941), streptomycin (1943), combination drugs, such as para-aminosalicylic acid (1944) and isoniazid (1952) into clinical practices contributed to a sharp decline in the death of patients affected by diseases such as pneumonia, influenza, and tuberculosis (8.2% per year in the USA) [5, 6].

The beginning of the modernized "antibiotic era" is linked with the names of renowned scientists Paul Ehrlich and Alexander Fleming. The idea by Paul Ehrlich, known as "magic bullet", selectively exerts its full action only on the infectious microbes and not on the host organism [7, 8]. Since its inception, this became the mainspring of drug discoveries for the last 60 years, where a massive amount of antibiotics have been manufactured and utilized for a wide variety of purposes [9]. Their bombastic production due to technological advances has led to an ever-increasing demand that resulted in non-prescription and off-labeled use. This oversaturation of the globe because of these toxic agents significantly contributed to the selection of resistant strains of microorganisms and their circulation in microbial populations throughout the terrain. This generates an unremitting selection pressure which is not a usual natural process, but a fabricated circumstance overlaid on the environment called Antimicrobial Resistance (AMR) [9]. Ergo, antimicrobial medicines turn out to be feeble and infections become harder or impossible to treat and also increased the probability of disease spread, stern ailment, at last, heading towards the end of life (https://www.who.int/news-room/fact-sheets/detail/antimicrobial-resistance).

ANTIQUITY OF ANTIBIOTIC EXPLORATION AND CONCOMITANT PROGRESS OF ANTIBIOTIC RESISTANCE

Since the introduction of the foremost effective antimicrobial in 1937 (sulphonamides), the maturation of peculiar mechanisms of resistance has haunted their medicinal application [9]. In the pre-antibiotic era, the presence of antimicrobials (such as artemisinin, a potent anti-malarial drug) [10] in many herbs from Traditional Chinese Medicine (TCM) could be thought of as a means of remedies (used for millennia) [11]. The discovery of such antimicrobial active components during ancient times might have enriched the depository of antimicrobials used by conventional medicine. Simultaneously, selective pressures forced by these antimicrobials through the deep-rooted past of TCM may be one of the components putting up to the aggregation of antibiotic resistance genes (ARGs) in our community [7].

For example, the late 1930s reported the resistance of Sulfonamide and the same mechanism operates even 70 years later also [9]. Even before the entry of penicillin into the market in 1943 as a therapeutic agent, penicillinase, which is of bacterial origin (discovered in 1940) was already identified [12]. With the excessive use of antibiotics, resistant strains (having drug inactivating capability) became widespread, thereafter, artificial studies were ventured to improve the chemical nature of penicillin to block cleavage by penicillinases (β-lactamases).

The streptomycin-resistant mutant strains of *M.tuberculosis* were detected to have risen during the treatment of the disease. In the mid-1950s, in Japan, the unanticipated identification of genetically transferable antibiotic resistance [13] changed the whole picture. Introduction of the concept of skeptical genetics, collections of ARGs could be propagated by bacterial conjugation mostly throughout the community of bacterial pathogens [14].

Over several decades, AMR caused severe infections that developed resistance and are incurable with available and new anti-microbial agents. The techniques like phylogenetic reconstruction help in revealing the history of these resistance genes and recommends the abiding existence of genes favoring resistance to varied antibiotics classes in the environment ahead of antibiotic ages [15]. The usage of molecular biology serves as the means of knowing the provenance and proliferation of drug resistance genes [16, 17].

In recent years, AMR has emerged as one of the key public health issues of the 21st century that menaces the effective avoidance and remedy of an ever-expanding range of infections caused by infectious agents that are no longer prone to the customary medicines used to cure them. The complication of AMR, specifically in the case of multi-resistant and pan-resistant bacteria (which are also called "superbugs"), requires urgent attention and solution. Also, the clinical interface of the medical pipeline of new antimicrobials is almost dry. In 2019, the World Health Organization (WHO) addressed the list of priority pathogens and identified 32 antibiotics in clinical development, of which only 6 were thought to be as innovative. Moreover, the inadequacy of access to quality anti-microbial remains a major concern. Antibiotic scarcities are striking nations of all levels of advancement and, principally, the medical management systems.

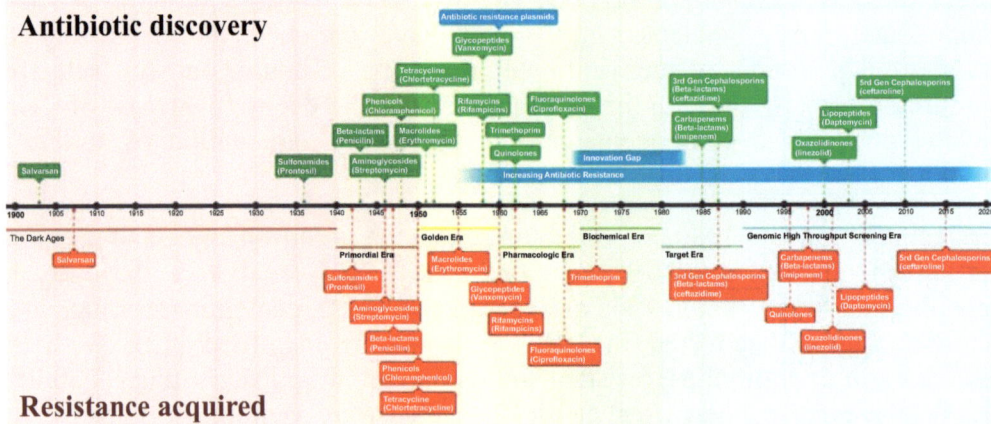

Fig. (1). Timeline showing antimicrobial discovery and acquired resistance for the century. All discoveries are the introduction of antibiotic can be depicted in green and all acquired resistance time-points can be observed in red. Different ages of antimicrobial inventions (Dark Age, golden era, *etc.*) are also shown in different background colors.

Fig. (**1**) shows the progression of discovery and resistance evolution for the main classes of antibiotics. The cost of AMR to social economies and their healthcare systems is serious as it disturbs the patients' productivity or their caretakers through extended hospital stays and the need for more costly and rigorous care [18]. Without efficient tools for prevention, ample treatment, and enhanced access to existing and new quality-assured anti-microbials, the number of people to whom treatment is not working or who die of infections will increase. Most of the advanced medical procedures, like surgery, including cesarean sections (1.2M women had a C-section in 2017) or hip replacements, cancer chemotherapy (around 650,000 people receive chemotherapy each year), organ transplantation (more than 33,000 transplants were performed in 2016), and chronic diseases treatment like diabetes (more than 30M) [19], asthma, and rheumatoid arthritis will become riskier [20].

No one can completely evade the threat of resistant infections. Encountered with this truth, the need for a plan to deter a flourishing global crisis in the medical sector is domineering [18] as it has the ability to affect society at any phase of life, may it be healthcare, agriculture industries, or veterinary, making it one of the most urgent global health concern [18]. Classes of antibiotics, their target and genes involved in resistance mechanism, which are important to deal with on a daily basis for drug resistance, are tabulated in Table **1**.

Table 1. Important classes of antibiotics and their candidate drug molecules along with targets resistance pathogens and genes involved in the resistance mechanism.

Class or Subclass	Target	WHO Critically Important Drug	Resistant Bacterium	Resistance Mechanism (Genes Involved)
Aminoglycosides	30S ribosomal subunit	Streptomycin (1943)	*M.tuberculosis*	Inactivation by bacterial enzymes, efflux pumps (Arm, aph, spd, ant, ade, acc, apw, rmt)
Carbapenems	Penicillin Binding proteins (inhibit the synthesis of peptidoglycan)	Imipenem (1985)	*K.pneumonia* (carbapenemase-producing) (1996)	Efflux, altered drug target due to hydrolysis (Ade, bla, mec, cme, mex)
Cephalosporins	Penicillin Binding proteins	Cefotaxime (1980)	*E.coli* (beta-lactamase-producing) (1983)	Efflux, drug target alteration, hydrolysis (Ade, mec, bla, mex, cme)
		Ceftazidime-avibactam (2015)	*K.pneumonia* (2015)	
Diarylquinolines	mycobacterial ATP synthase	Bedaquiline (2004)	*M.tuberculosis* (2014)	-
Glycopeptides	Peptidoglycan units	Vancomycin (1958)	*E.faecium* (Plasmid-mediated) (1988) *S.aureus* (2002)	Modification of the drug target, increased drug efflux
Lipopeptides	Cell membrane	Daptomycin (2003)	*S.aureus* (methicillin-resistant) (2004)	Antibiotic efflux (*Bcr*)
Macrolides	50S ribosomal subunit	Azithromycin (1980)	*N.gonorrhoeae* (2011)	Glycosylation, phosphorylation, hydrolysis, efflux, drug target modification (Ere, mph, cfr, erm, mef, msr)
Oxazolidinones	50S ribosomal subunit	Linezolid (1990s)	*E.faecium*	Drug efflux, drug target alteration or inactivation (Erm, inu, inu, vga, cfr, msr)

(Table 1) cont.....

Class or Subclass	Target	WHO Critically Important Drug	Resistant Bacterium	Resistance Mechanism (Genes Involved)
Penicillins	Penicillin Binding proteins	Penicillin (1941)	*S.aureus* (1942) *S.pneumonia* (1967) *N.gonorrhoeae* (Penicillinase-producing) (1976)	Efflux, altered drug target due to hydrolysis (Ade, bla, mec, cme, mex)
		Methicillin (1960)	*S.aureus* (1960)	Efflux, altered drug target due to hydrolysis (Ade, bla, mec, cme, mex)
Pleuromutilins	50S ribosome	Retapamulin (2007)	-	Change in the drug target, drug efflux (Sal, vga, cfr, isa)
Polymyxins	the outer cell membrane of gram-negative bacteria	Colistin (1949)	*E.coli* (2015)	Drug target modification, enhanced drug efflux (mgr, pmr AB)
Quinolones	Topoisomerase II and IV	Ciprofloxacin (1985)	*N.gonorrhoeae* (2007)	Altered drug target, inactivation of the drug by bacterial enzymes, drug efflux (Aac (6′), qnr, gyr A, oqx, parC)
Rifamycins	RNA Polymerase	Rifabutin (1975)	*H.pylori* (1990s)	Drug efflux
Streptogramins	50S ribosomal subunit	Dalfopristin (1999)	*E.faecium*	Change in a target of the drug, efflux or drug inactivation by bacterial enzymes (Erm, Vgb, Vga, Isa, cfr, vat)

Class or Subclass	Target	WHO Critically Important Drug	Resistant Bacterium	Resistance Mechanism (Genes Involved)
Sulfonamides	dihydropteroate synthase (DHPS) in the folic acid pathway	Trimethoprim (1960s)	*Enterococcal* species	Altered drug target, increased efflux of antibiotics (acr, sul, dhfr, bpr-opc)
Tetracyclines	30S ribosomal subunit	Tigecycline (2005)	*E.faecalis* (2007)	Drug efflux, drug modification by bacterial enzymes, altered binding site (*Otr*, *tet*)

THE SCENARIO OF DRUG RESISTANCE: GLOBAL AND INDIAN PERSPECTIVE

AMR is a crucial global issue akin to climate change threatening both peoples' health and global development. Infections caused by AMR pathogens cause a significant menace to health-care and human financing. If this is left rampant, it will likely lead to 10 million deaths yearly by 2050 [21].

Most of the fatality is due to multidrug-resistant (MDR) bacteria like *K.pneumoniae*, *E.faecium*, *S.aureus*, *E.coli*, *S.pneumoniae*, and *P.aeruginosa*. Pneumonia kills almost 10 lakhs children annually (below five years), and approximately 4.45 lakhs of kids could be rescued with the supply of antibiotics for community-acquired pneumococcal infections. When proper medication is accessible, first-line antibiotic treatments are still comparably economical, but newer antibiotics (needed for treating resistant infections) may be inaccessible in remote areas [22, 23].

The Centre for Disease Control and Prevention (CDC) predicted that in the United States (US), fatality from infections caused by antimicrobial-resistant is reported at 35,000 deaths yearly [24], with heavy production losses estimated at US$ 35 billion [25].

The AMR report by the European Union commission claims that, in Europe, the annual hospital fatality rate is estimated at around 33,000 with costs totaling greater than €1.5 billion [26] whereas AMR is mostly neglected in Nepal due to improper implementation and execution of the law, other public health preferences, and misuse of general antimicrobials in humans and animals [27].

Like many other developing countries, Libya also faces the problem of antimicrobial agents misuse (can be purchased without any prescription from pharmacies). Also, methicillin-resistant *S.aureus* (MRSA) was reported at a high prevalence rate (54–68%) in the last decade from patients with surgical wound infections and burns [28].

In Pakistan, antibiotic consumption between the years 2000 and 2015 has increased by 65% (*i.e.*) the country observed a surge from 16.2-19.6 DDD per 1,000 people per day. Due to extensive drug abuse, MDR is also rising steadily. It is the third-highest consumer of antibiotics among the 76 low- and middle-income countries (LMICs). In addition to this, Pakistan is also playing a part in the evolution of far more resistant mutated genes than their pioneer form of the microbes [29].

Multidrug-resistant typhoidal (up to 89% isolates tested) and non-typhoidal *Salmonella* infections (50 to 75% isolates tested) [30, 31] are on the rise in Sub-Saharan Africa.

In India, the burden of infectious diseases and antimicrobial resistance rates is among the topmost in the world. Reports showed that ludicrous use of antimicrobial agents has led to a hike in the AMR levels [32], including the biggest problem of multidrug-resistant tuberculosis (MDR-TB). Perturbingly, high resistance to newer antimicrobials (since its introduction in 2010) such as faropenem and carbapenems has been reported among Gram-negative and Gram-positive bacteria. Regional studies also report a higher AMR among infectious agents such as *S.typhi*, *Pseudomonas*, *Shigella,* and *Acinetobacter.* Aminopenicillins resistance against *Acinetobacter baumannii* has reached almost 100% in India (Fig. **2**).

In India, every year, over 56,000 newborn babies die [33] due to sepsis (at least 1.7M adults develop sepsis each year [19]). This is caused by pathogens that are resistant to first-line antibiotics [22, 34, 35]. The environment, especially the water bodies due to demographic and civilization factors prevalent have also contributed to the presence of resistant genes or organisms. Imprudent use of antimicrobials and meager wastewater treatment are important factors in AMR. Improper disposal of livestock and sludge use in agriculture contributors to AMR in other countries but India [36].

As of now, there are only few antibiotics like Carbapenems, Aminoglycosides, polymyxins and Glycylcuclines that are effective against *E.coli* infections (Fig. **3**).

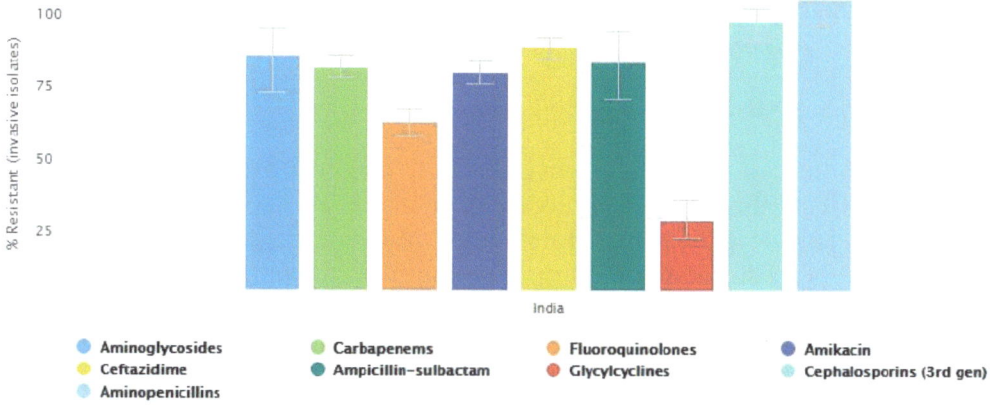

Fig. (2). Prevalence of drug resistance in *A.baumannii* in India. Aminopenicillins resistance level has reached the 100% followed by 3rd generation cephalosporins (~90%).

Antibiotic Resistance of *Escherichia coli*

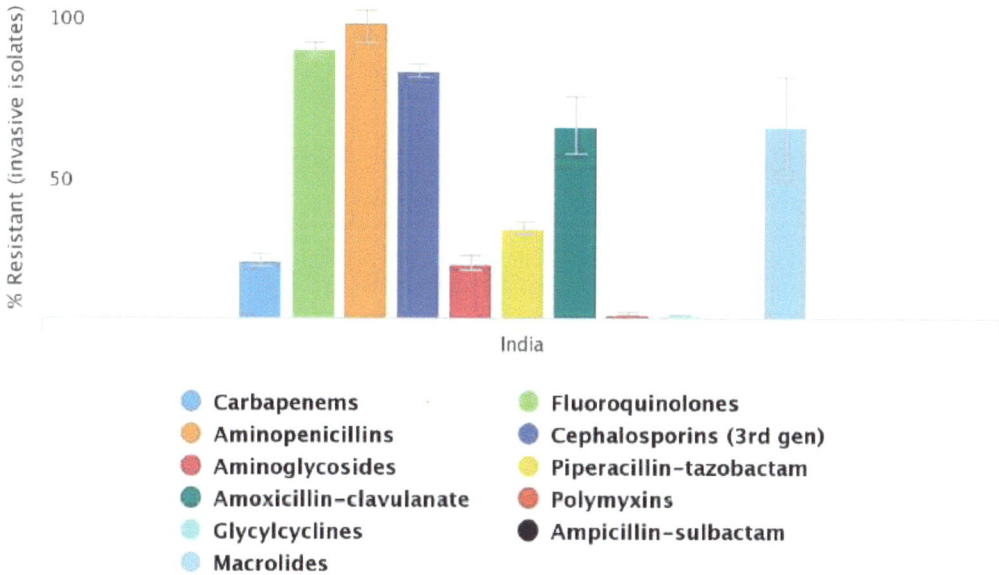

Fig. (3). This figure shows the till date data for antibiotic resistance in India. Resistance against Aminopenicillins is touching the level of 100% resistance followed by the fluoroquinolones resistance.

A. baumannii and *E. coli*, and *K. pneumoniae* showed more than 70% resistance to the Broad-spectrum antibiotics such as fluoroquinolones, and 3rd generation cephalosporin (Fig. **3**), and above 50% in *P.aeruginosa* [37]. In case of carbapenem (one of the last-resort antibiotics to treat serious bacterial infections in humans) the highest resistance was noticed in *A. baumannii* (70.9%), followed by 56.6% in *K. pneumoniae*, 46.8% in *P. aeruginosa*, and 16.2% in *E. coli* [37].

SUPERBUGS AND DRUG RESISTANCE

A superbug refers to a pathogen (includes both bacterial and fungal strains) that frequently affects the living creatures like humans, animals, and crops and has formed a resistance against multiple drugs. Microbes that generate antibiotics naturally are also resistant to them. As antibiotics were discovered to treat infections caused by pathogens widely, simultaneously, these pathogens have also started to explore new ways to their survival [38]. The ESKAPE (*E.faecium, S. aureus*, K. pneumoniae, A. baumannii, P. aeruginosa, and Enterobacter spp.) [39] group of organisms is considered 'Superbugs' as they are divergently becoming resistant to all the classes of antibiotics used so far (Fig. **4**). After MDR and XDR (extensively drug-resistant), a new classification has already emerged called PDR (pan-drug resistant) which is not at all getting killed by any of the drug molecules discovered till now [40].

Fig. (4). ABR graph for *E. faecium*. Aminopenicillins resistance is commonly predominant in almost every shown country. Fluoroquinolones and aminoglycosides resistance is in advanced stages in India.

Fig. (**5**) depicts the antibiotic resistance data of *Staphalococous aureus*, where most of the world population has hand full of drugs that works against this pathogen except India.

Fig. (5). ABR profile for *S.aureaus*. As observed, almost all drugs are non-functional in India against this organism.

In recent years, the rise of colistin-resistant, carbapenem-resistant *K.pneumoniae* (CRKP), which is grouped under the class of 'critical pathogen' by the WHO, has been one of the major public threat worldwide. The CRKP isolates are extremely multidrug-resistant and have the usual tendency to cause uropathogenic infections, chronic liver infections, and respiratory tract diseases leaving the subject with a few or no treatment options [41]. Worldwide, this pathogen is almost resistant to all groups of antibiotics available till date (Fig. **6**).

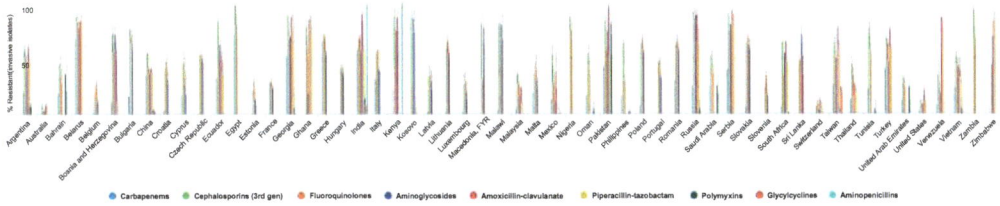

Fig. (6). ABR illustration for *K.pneumonia*. Almost all continents are covered with the attack of this resistant organism which is resistant against almost all drugs.

Similarly, Carbapenem-resistant *A.baumannii* has been declared by the WHO as a 'Critical' pathogen immediately requiring novel therapeutic strategies [42] as almost all the drugs have become ineffective (Fig. **7**). The in-hospital fatality rate in subjects with bloodstream infections caused by *A. baumannii* has attained nearly 25% of the total cases.

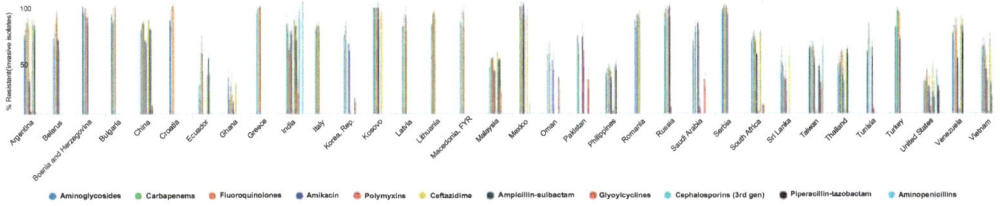

Fig. (7). ABR profile for *A.baumanni* showing fluoroquinolones, prevailing the countries throughout followed by third-generation Cephalosporins.

P. aeruginosa is the first ranking candidate in the race of 'superbugs'. It exhibits decreasing susceptibility to almost all antibiotics due to low outer membrane permeability linked to adaptive mechanisms and can promptly accomplish clinical resistance [43]. Multi-channel outbreaks of Metallo-β-lactamase-producing *P.aeruginosa* resistant to carbapenems were identified from 1992 to 1994 in Japan [44]. Aminopenicillin and cephalosporin resistance has reached almost 100% in India (Fig. **8**).

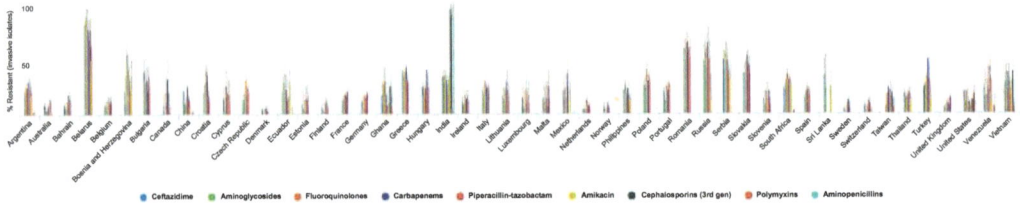

Fig. (8). ABR map for *P.aeruginosa*. The highest level of resistance against Aminopenicillins and cephalosporins can be observed in India and mostly all drugs show less susceptibility against *P.aeruginosa* in Bulgaria.

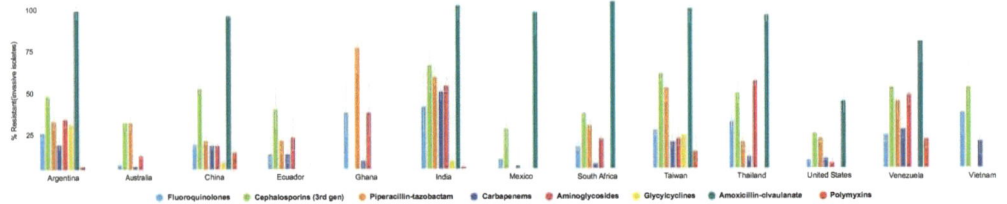

Fig. (9). ABR profiling for Enterobacter aerogenes/cloacae. Clearly defined Amoxicillin-clavulanate resistance can be observed in all the depicted nations except Vietnam.

In most of the countries like India, China, South Africa, Thailand, Taiwan, Mexico, and Argentina, *E. aerogenes* shows increased resistance to Amoxicillin-clavulanate (Fig. **9**).

Pedobacter spp. (isolated from soils, chilled food, drinking water, compost, fish, and other extreme environments) are intrinsically resistant to most antibiotics. Around 6-8% of their total protein-encoding genes encode a diverse set of putative ARGs, including β-lactamases (enzymes highly abundant in all strains of *Pedobacter*) thereby making them environmental superbugs [45].

There is an alarming increase in rare opportunistic microbial infections around the globe. *M. morganii* is one of its kind, whose opportunism is being highly reported worldwide. This has the capability of accumulating both intrinsic and acquired MDR genes, resulting in increased sickness and fatality rates for pre-and post-operation *M. morganii* infections and complicating its treatment [46].

MOLECULAR MECHANISMS OF THE RESISTANCE

Though various types of antimicrobial resistance mechanisms have been claimed in bacteria, they can be majorly categorized as:

Decreased Antibiotics Permeability

The presence of a thick layer of mycolic acid serves as causes a major permeability barrier to most antibiotics. This inhibits the entry of most drugs [47]. Also, porin present in the outer membrane of gram-negative bacteria imparts a major permeability obstacle to a huge lot of antibiotics.

Depravity of Antibacterials by Bacterial Enzymes

The bacterial β-lactamases have the potential to degrade β-lactam antibiotics. This is achieved by disrupting the β-lactam ring of the antibiotics. Also, some antibiotics can be disrupted by adding specific groups to their chemical structure. For example, chloramphenicol possesses a hydroxyl group that can be acetylated by the addition of acetyl-CoA. By the addition of acetyl-CoA, phosphate, and adenylyl group, Aminoglycosides can also be degraded and these reactions are carried out by acetyltransferases, phosphor-transferases, and adenyl transferases respectively [48, 49].

Enhanced Antimicrobials Efflux

Numerous bacterial species like *S. aureus*, E. coli, and *P. aeruginosa* possess efflux pumps. These pumps actively release drugs thereby reducing the bactericidal concentration of the antimicrobials. These pumps are actively involved in the evolution and rise of resistance against innumerable antibiotics especially against tetracyclines, aminoglycosides, and sulfonamides [50].

Alternative Pathway Usage by Bacteria

Few microbes can change the usual pathway that has been inhibited by specific antimicrobials. For example, a phenomenon known as competitive antagonism where some bacteria rather than synthesizing folic acid, uses the preordain folic acid, which is inhibited by sulfonamides [51].

Drug Target Modification

Resistance development against the drug in bacteria can also occur when their initial binding target is altered. Modification in the ribosomal binding sites against macrolides and phenolics drugs leads to a drastic reduction in antimicrobial activity [52]. Also, *E.coli* possessing the *mcr*-1 gene can adjoin a compound to the outside of the cell wall so that colistin drug can't get into it [19].

OTHER FACTORS CAUSING ANTIMICROBIAL DRUG RESISTANCE

Self-medication (Drug Abuse)

As quoted by Alexander Fleming "the ignorant man may easily under-dose himself and by exposing his microbes to non-lethal quantities of the drug make them resistant" [53]. Self-medication is defined as the selection and use of medicines by people to treat self-identified illnesses or related symptoms. It is considered to be one of the major factors contributing to drug resistance [54] and directly related to the risk of using inappropriate drugs [55], thereby, concealing the symptoms of primary disease, and the development of resistance to that drug in the longer run [56]. In the Southeast Asian region, antibiotics are bought and used without any doctor's prescription. The key reasons behind these self-medication antibiotics were based on earlier positive experience (34.4%) and the disease or the symptoms being not serious enough to seek a medical practitioner (25.7%). Wound infection (17.9%) and sore throat (13.9%) are the most self-identified problems that required self-medication. 84.1% of those who self-medicated used amoxicillin at least once in their life [57]. Fig. (**10**) represents the usage of antibiotics worldwide (Defined daily doses/1000 population), in the year 2015.

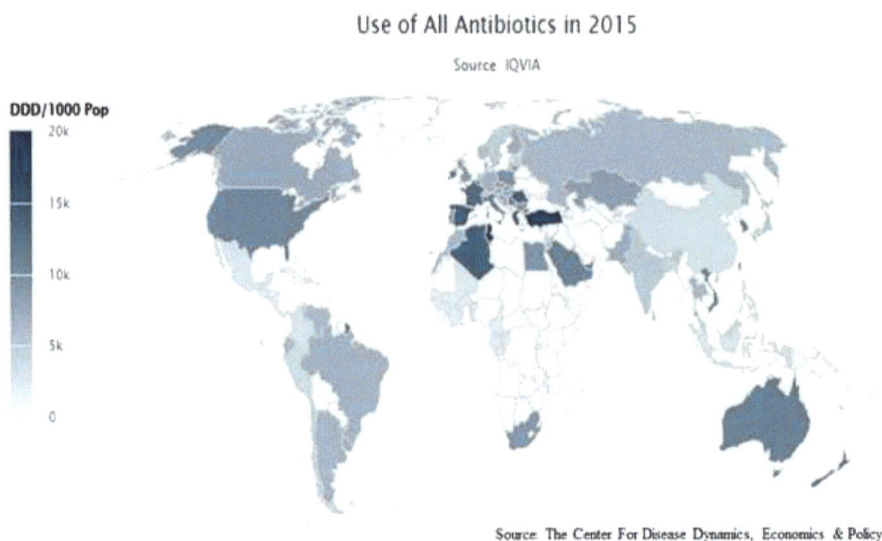

Use of All Antibiotics in 2015

Source IQVIA

Source: The Center For Disease Dynamics, Economics & Policy

Fig. (10). Map shows the usage of all antibiotics in the year 2015. Dark blue areas represent the intake of more than 20,000 defined daily doses of all available antibiotics. Turkey used 18,095 DDD/1000 population followed by Tunisia with 17,572 DDD/1000.

Evolution and Transmission of Resistance Genes

Microbes have a very deep-root history in this world, due to random mutation (because of strong evolutionary selection pressures) over trillions of generations, microbes have accommodated to nature, partly by initializing genes that code for the phenomenon of resistance to multiple menaces like human interventions, heavy metals, naturally occurring and synthetic antimicrobial compounds) [58, 59]. Importantly, certain microbes can horizontally relocate the genes coding for the mechanisms of resistance to other pathogenic organisms [60]. It is also transmitted between humans just like other pathogens *viz* skin contact, air-borne transmission, sexual transfer, orofecal route, vector transmission, and contact with the infected fluid of the body, along with contaminated food and water [61, 62].

Travel, Migration, and Trade

Bacterial resistance to all classes of antibiotics *i.e.* first-line, second-line, and last-resort is growing steeply (though trends and rates differ by an organism, location, and antibiotic) [63]. The spread of drug resistance worldwide is highly accelerated by increased travel, migration, and trade (by providing resistant bacteria to spread faster than ever) [64, 65]. Travelers from developed countries, visiting LMICs (South Asian Indian subcontinent- highest risk), often acquire drug-resistant bacteria (mainly extended-spectrum β-lactamase-producing Enterobacteriaceae). Also, MDR enteric infections in travelers (refugees, pilgrimages, and medical tourists) from *Campylobacter spp., Salmonella spp., and Shigella spp.,* are at spike [17]. MDR-TB is more prevalent among migrants than the native inhabitants (in low-incidence countries in Europe) in which, a significant proportion is due to reactivation of the latent infection. Existing processes and policies lack the capacity to prevent or mitigate adverse health effects [66 - 68].

Population Mediated Pollution

AMR has emerged as a natural process, but it can also be fabricated by the exposure of antimicrobials in clinical and veterinary medicine [69]. The prevalence of antibiotic-resistant E.coli and enterococci was found in fecal samples of a healthy population. The overall consumption of antibiotics in both Newfoundland and Greece was more than three times higher compared with that of The Netherlands. In Newfoundland, the lowest prevalence of drug-resistant *E.coli* was found and was significant for oxytetracycline, cefazolin, and trimethoprim [70]. A hike in population density through urbanization leads to many occasions for interpersonal contact, promoting the spread of resistant bacteria and its genes, and may contribute to an important part in the propagation of antibiotic resistance [70, 71]. Fecal pollution testing is used to detect the presence of resistance genes in densely populated regions where environmental selection also plays a major role. Areas near antibiotics manufacturing are more prone to resistance genes [72].

Climatic Change

Every 10°C rise in temperature along with growing population density was associated with an increase in antibiotic resistance of common pathogens like *E.coli (4.2%), K.pneumoniae* (2.2%), and *S.aureus* (2.7%) [73]. The associations between the climatic changes and antibiotic resistance are consistent across most classes of antibiotics and may be strengthening in the longer run. The temperature effect on clinically relevant phenotypes has been exhibited by *A.baumannii* at 37°C and 28°C. Bio-film formation on plastic surfaces was escalated at 28°C, while surface-associated motility was remarkably reduced at 28°C. Also, at 28°C, enhanced susceptibility to trimethoprim-sulfamethoxazole and reduced sensitivity to aztreonam was observed [74]. Both temperature and antibiotics, act on similar cellular functions. Therefore, mutations conferring resistance to temperature stress can confer resistance to antibiotics and *vice-versa* [75], a phenomenon known as cross-protection or collateral resistance [75]. To fully understand this, there is a need for a multi-scale and multidisciplinary approach that completely records and examines the effects of temperature [75].

An appropriate or inappropriate use of an antibiotic exerts a selection pressure that accelerates the emergence of resistance. Intake of antibiotics is rising globally, especially in economically lower and middle countries. Besides the burden of infectious disease, antibiotic consumption by humans is also driven by environmental, behavioral, economic, and structural factors. Also, expanded insurance coverage, decision fatigue, increased physician density, and patient demand have lead to the consumption of (irrelevant) antibiotics or antibiotic prescribing. Antibiotic use is also correlated with the season, which increases in the winter with the increase in the incidence of infectious disease [76 - 80].

Antibiotic Use in Agriculture and Animals

Agriculture and food animals are crucial players in AMR sources as they are susceptible to the large volume of antibiotics [81]. Transmission of resistance takes place through contact with people working with animals, food chain, and manure-contaminated environments. Antibiotics are largely used in mastitis cases. Drug termination periods are hardly observed and the prevalence of milk contaminated with milk antibiotics has been reported. The recent report of plasmid-mediated colistin resistance genes found in raw food, slaughtered pigs, and humans bring into light the risk of transmission from animals to humans [82].

SURVEILLANCE MECHANISM FOR ANTIMICROBIAL RESISTANCE

The implication of acquiring and utilizing the information regarding the impact of drug resistance on our ecosystem needs to be re-considered for the design of a better surveillance mechanism. AMR surveillance provides an opportunity to tackle the burden of AMR and the development of new working strategies for control and prevention. The co-development of AMR surveillance strategies is essential both in humans and animals. However, several key elements make the data comparisons between AMR monitoring systems difficult. In the current scenario, AMR surveillance relies solely on *in-vitro* susceptibility methods. Nonetheless, strategic harmonization across programs and the limitation of genetic information of AMR remain the major drawbacks of these phenotypic methods [83].

With the increase in MDR and XDR cases throughout the globe, detection of resistant strains is routinely performed using usual phenotypic methods. Molecular ways are often used in addition to phenotypic methods in detecting the underlying genetic mechanism(s) for drug resistance. Some of the most common molecular methods for the detection of AMR currently in use are PCR, DNA microarray, whole-genome sequencing and metagenomics, and matrix-assisted laser desorption ionization-time of flight mass spectrometry (MALDI-ToF). The pros and cons of these methods vary, mostly in the context of implementing them for routine testing activities on a global scale [84].

The futuristic AMR surveillance is prevailing forward towards genotypic detection and these molecular analysis methods are shown to be a wealth of crucial information. However, it is a distant reality that these molecular techniques have become a common mode of routine diagnostics. This infers that phenotypic testing remains necessary in the detection of emerging resistant bacteria, new resistance mechanisms, and trends of AMR in near future too [83]. The critical point to note is that there is still a huge backlog of knowledge and research data on different food-borne pathogens as well as several antibiotics families such as macrolides and quinolones. The novel combination of MALDI-TOF MS and whole-genome sequencing could be the future for AMR diagnosis in food-originated pathogens [85].

The genetic and ecological aspects of AMR are interrelated. An example of this is mutualistic associations among microbes like biofilms can both serve as a hurdle to antibiotic penetration and also act as a breeding ground for horizontal exchange of ARGs [86]. Technological advances such as next-generation sequencing are expanding our capacities to detect and study AMR. The AMR surveillance mechanisms and methods have developed from age-old antimicrobial susceptibility testing (AST) to recent deep-learning methods. Boolchandani and group focused on sequencing-based resistance discovery and they also discussed tools and databases used in AMR studies [87].

The rapid ongoing increase in the availability of high-density genomic data for a myriad array of bacteria leads to the development of algorithms that could utilize this information to predict new phenotypic targets of AMR pathways that will help solve this issue clinically. To understand the connections between DNA variation and phenotypic AMR, Kim, and the group [88] developed a new in-silico tool VAMPr, to derive gene ortholog-based sequence features for protein variants to build accurate models to predict whole-genome sequencing-based AMR. The association models made by VAMPr confirmed known genetic antibiotic resistance trends and mechanisms, such as β-lactamase Klebsiella pneumoniae carbapenemase (blaKPC) and carbapenem resistance consistent with the accurate nature of the approach. The prediction models have achieved high accuracies through internal nested cross-validation and external clinical data. The VAMPr variant detection method will be a valuable tool for AMR research with the potential for clinical applicability [88].

In the continuation, the description of single-cell technologies that were developed to hasten the AST of infectious pathogens cannot be ignored. The concluding address shows the potential of recently developed rapid diagnostic systems as point-of-care (POC) diagnostic tools and the challenges to adapt them at the current status of rapid and POC diagnostic systems for AMR [21].

Although the prevalence, cause, and effect of drug resistance are well studied, the rate of transmission is poorly understood. Bennani and team [89] reviewed the already reported evidence on the links between antimicrobial use (AMU) in the food chain and AMR on the organism level. The clear link between AMU in animals and the occurrence of resistance in these animals has been shown. Although, there is a scarcity of evidence of the benefits of a reduction in AMU in animals on the prevalence of resistant bacteria in humans. The presence of resistant bacterial strains in the human food supply chain and Microbial genome sequencing also doesn't provide any link that could be predefined. A high level of Research and monitoring of AMR in an integrated manner is essential for a better understanding of the biology and the dynamics of AMR [89]. AMR Research has prevalently focused on genetic exchange phenomenon and abiotic environmental constraints, leaving important points of microbial ecology still unresolved.

The reduction in childhood fatality has been noted as an effect of large randomized controlled trials investigating azithromycin mass drug administration (MDA) for trachoma control. This drive suggested that targeted surveillance is necessary for focusing on a genotypic approach to overcome the limitations of resistance surveillance in indicator bacteria [90].

The drug resistance surveillance should satisfy some conditions to make the search better and efficient. AMS team composition, infrastructure requirements for AMR surveillance, and susceptibility patterns to report; data stratification strategies; frequency of reporting; surveillance in high-risk hospital units, long-term care, and veterinary settings; and surveillance data from other countries. Twenty such guidelines of AMR surveillance should be implemented as part of an

AMS program. These procedures should be mandated to settings outside the acute-care institutions, such as long-term care, outpatient, and veterinary. Without suitable surveillance, the implementation of AMS policies cannot contribute majorly to the fight against MDR pathogens and may even worsen the burden of adverse situations from such interventions [91].

In the course of the development of antimicrobial peptides (AMP) as an effective treatment strategy, AST stands as an important part in the process of the identification and optimization of candidate AMP. Highly physiologically relevant AST will allow better perseverance of preclinical activity of the drug candidates and recognition of lead compounds. A crucial concern is the efficacy of AMP in biological matrices depicting the sites of infection, like blood, plasma, biofilms, serum, urine, lung bronchiolar sputum, *etc.*, as this will likely be more anticipative of clinical efficacy. Also, specific AST for different target microbes may help to better predict the efficiency of AMP in particular infections [92].

SUBDUE ANTIMICROBIAL RESISTANCE

Drug discovery has suffered from the inadequacy of exploitable binding sites in bacteria, leading to the slow emergence of truly novel drugs. Modification of existing antimicrobial agents to achieve theoretical benefits is often seen as commercially safer. In humans, there are many ways to assist this goal, including the implementation and adherence to guidelines given by international organizations such as the World Health Organization and the Centres for Disease Control and Prevention, as well as through the implementation of rapid diagnostic tests for AMR. Additionally, infection prevention activities also need to be put forth to reduce the need for treatment [81].

New Targets to Address Current Drug Resistance

Raetz Pathway

The increasing problem of AMR (especially in Gram-negative bacterial pathogens) and MDR necessitates the characterization of new antibiotic targets. As the study of Lipids requires more technical challenges than other biological molecules (nucleic acids, proteins, and carbohydrates), it has received a lesser research focus [93]. The Raetz pathway (also known as Lipid A biosynthesis pathway) is vital for most Gram-negative bacteria (for its survival and fitness) and also comprises several novel targets. In Gram-negative bacteria, lipid A forms the membrane anchor of lipopolysaccharide (LPS). This LPS forms the outer leaflet of the outer membrane and protects the bacteria from environmental stressors [94 - 100]. The novel target proteins of Raetz pathway are, (in number starting from) LpxA, LpxC, LpxD, LpxH (LpxI and LpxG, analog of LpxH), LpxB, LpxK, kdtA, LpxL to the final LpxM (Fig. **11**). The initial building block for these enzymes to work is UDP-diacyl-GlcN which transformed into Lipid A after the completion of bio-action of the 9th enzyme (LpxM). The rate-limiting step in this whole pathway is the second step catalyzed by the enzyme LpxC. In the fourth step, UDP-diacyl-GlcN is hydrolyzed by LpxH to form lipid X. Depending on the bacterial species, the formation of lipid X is mediated by either LpxH or its analog. These enzymes are peripheral membrane proteins, and their reactions occur in the vicinity of the membrane. LpxH (UDP-diacylglucosamine pyrophosphohydrolase) which has less sequence conservation with other bacterial species and lacks a mammalian homolog promises to be an excellent drug target for the development of novel antibiotics [101 - 105].

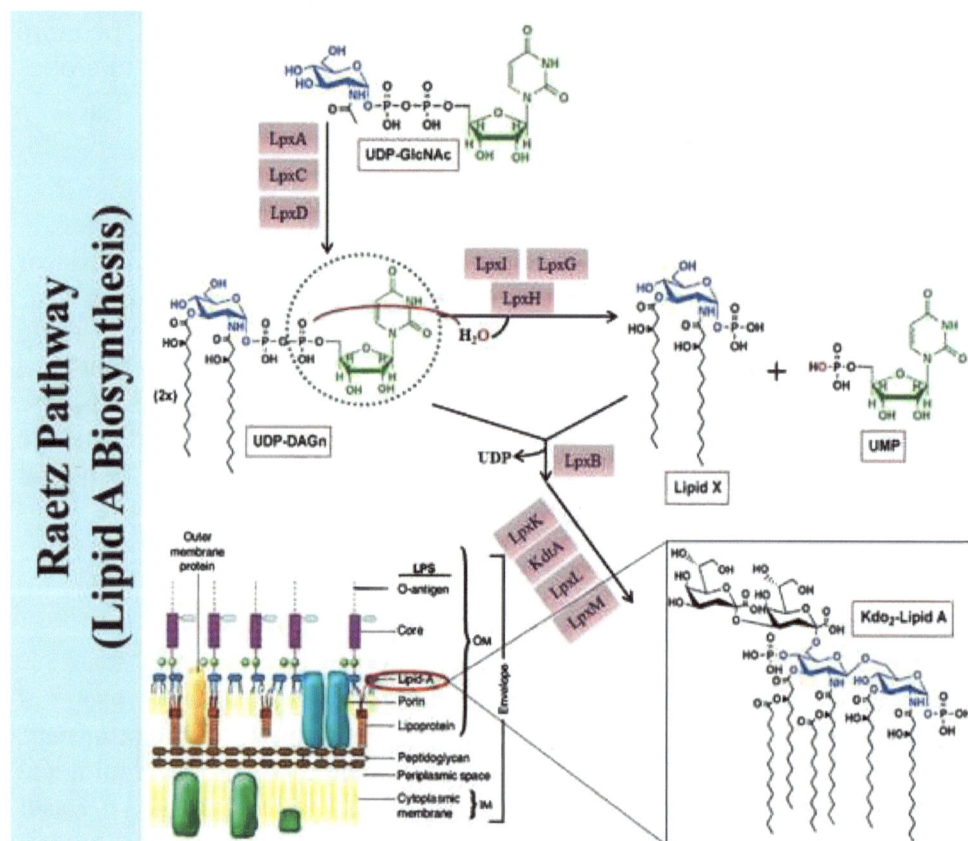

Fig. (11). Raetz Pathway reperesentation for Lipid A biosynthesis. 9 crucial enzymes (LpxA, LpxC, LpxD, LpxH, LpxB, LpxK, KdtA, LpxL, LpxM) work together catalysing each step of Lipid A sysnthesis.

At Merck Research Laboratories, L-573,655 was selected (screening of compounds) [106] and was tested for sensitivity against all nine enzymes of Raetz Pathway, in which it was known to inhibit LpxC (inhibition constant: 24 μM).

Then, threonyl-hydroxamate-containing compounds were developed (like CHIR-090) with antibacterial activity similar to that of ciprofloxacin [107]. Based on their interactions with LpxC, the inhibitor was further made potent by attaching bulky groups to threonyl-hydroxamate (*e.g.* LPC-051) [108].

Other New Antimicrobial Targets

The majority of current antibiotics have the same target. The range of these targets is limited to the components of the translational machinery, cell wall biosynthesis, majority, and some other cellular processes. With the extensive help of genome sequencing, it's possible to implement the idea of magic, with essential targets exactly at the molecular level [109]. The comparison of metabolic pathways in pathogenic and commensal bacteria helps in identifying the novel drug/target combinations in pathogens [110] (in the suppression of key virulence factor, type III secretion system [111], and in the inhibition of the QseC-mediated activation of virulence gene expression in many pathogens [112]). Already approved drugs, designed for a different purpose may find their application as antimicrobials (BPH-652, a phosphonosulfonate, initially tested for cholesterol-reducing activity) [113].

Other potential targets include cell division [114], bacterial two-component signal transduction [115], quorum sensing [116], fatty acid biosynthesis [117], biosynthesis of aminoacyl-tRNAs [118], and proton motive force [119]. Also, by targeting AMR mechanisms like β-lactamases, efflux pumps to regain the efficiency of antibiotics [120, 121]. Also, the intervention strategies aiming at biological networks might assist in discovering new antibacterial therapies [122]. Combination therapy *i.e.*, coupling antibiotics with an antibiotic-enhancing phage has been proven to be a promising idea [123].

Implementation of Antimicrobial Stewardship Programs

Faced with many defense mechanisms against all antimicrobials, it's time for a rejuvenate respect for the relationship between microorganisms, antimicrobials, and resistance processes and drivers. Today, in the human administration of antibiotics, this is called stewardship. Antimicrobial stewardship (AMS) is also one of the recently devised methods for better AMR surveillance and policy-making. It has appeared as a systematic path to optimize antimicrobial usage and slash AMR [124]. AMS explains a coherent set of actions that guarantee optimal use of antimicrobials to increase patient outcomes while curbing the danger of adverse events like AMR. Though this concept was introduced in the 1980s, it had no validation until a randomized controlled study showed that antibiotic use could be notably decreased without adverse outcomes [125, 126]. Since then, it has heightened and developed into a formalized, prospective, multi-disciplinary program. Active interventions, such as, optimizing dose regime, discontinuing superfluous antibiotics, and abate from broad-spectrum to pathogen-directed therapies, have been shown to deflate price, toxicity and refrain from the selection of resistant species [127 - 129]. AMS programs in hospitals are an essential component of national action plans for AMR and have been shown to reduce AMR significantly. A proper protocol has been developed in all countries to set up and implement a hospital AMS program. This program will help healthcare professionals optimally design and implement their actions [124].

To support the implementation of AMS programs, WHO developed a draft toolkit for the health care system and conducted a study in Malawi, the Federated States of Micronesia, Bhutan, and Nepal to acquire local input on toolkit content and implementation of AMS programs. This descriptive qualitative study involved semi-structured interviews with the facility- and national-level stakeholders. Respondents recognized AMS as a priority and anticipated the draft toolkit as a much-required document to further AMS program implementation. Facilitators for achieving AMS included clinical staff engagement and strong national and facility leadership. Inadequate regulations for prescription antibiotic sales, lack of human and financial resources, and insufficient AMS training were the obstruction faced. The AMS toolkit was considered to be an essential asset as countries and health care sectors came forward to implement it [124, 130]. Though efforts have been made to encourage AMS internationally, this is still limited to acute care settings and tertiary centers. However, to optimize future benefits, such programs must be productive in all healthcare settings. Stewardship practices should not be restricted to antimicrobials used for treatment, should also include those used for prophylaxis. The role of good stewardship can be crippled when attention is highly directed to seemingly more concrete strategies such as reinforcing the pipeline of new antibiotics.

Non-Prescription Antibiotics

Access to non-prescription antimicrobial worldwide [131], inappropriately low antimicrobial doses [132 - 134], and evidence for the use of expired drugs [135 - 137] are associated with camouflaging the underlying infection and a contributor to increasing AMR. In Korea [138] and Chile [139], improved regulation of non-prescription antibiotics has reduced the resistance status. The challenges in changing this practice lie not only in implementing legislation that will avoid the use of over-the-counter antibiotics but increased awareness via educational interventions.

Reducing Antibiotic Use in Agriculture and Animals

For over 60 years, antibiotics have been used in agriculture, veterinary medicine, and animal husbandry to prevent, control and treat infections, which serve as a reservoir of ARGs [140 - 143]. The first country to ban antimicrobial use as growth promoters were Sweden followed by Denmark and Germany. The implementation of a European Union-wide ban occurred in 2006 [144]. However, in the majority of the world, widespread antimicrobial growth promoters occur. Efforts have been made by some countries, like the US, to rule out the use of antibiotics in animal feeds. Raising and regulating support and awareness amongst farmers, food producers, and retailers have taken place; still, more to be done globally [145]. Options like ensuring proper training, establishing standardized global surveillance of antibiotic use and resistance, cautious use of antibiotics, using phage therapy (the neutralization of food-borne pathogens in animals [146] and control of plant pathogens [147]), widening the vaccine range available for veterinary use, and using predatory bacteria in combating pathogenic bacteria [148, 149] for helping the concerns of the farming society while lowering their antimicrobial use.

Vaccination

With an estimated 11 million days of antibiotic treatment, the potential reduction in antibiotic use attributable to vaccination is considerable. This could be bypassed by the introduction of the pneumococcal vaccine universally [22]. Influenza can be exactly predicted only using the antibiotic sales data and an estimated 20% reduction in influenza would reduce antibiotic prescribing by 8% in the US. A universal vaccination program in Ontario, Canada, was found to decrease influenza-associated antibiotic prescribing by 64% [150, 151]. Up to 40% of influenza-associated secondary bacterial infection cases (that require hospitalization) can be averted by applying Influenza vaccination [152, 153]. A similar reduction pattern in antibiotic usage is likely to be achieved by the introduction of vaccines for bacterial diarrheal and viral infections, such as cholera and rotavirus [154, 155].

Incidence of infection with both multidrug- and penicillin-resistant strains of S.pneumoniae in the US has reduced by more than 50% after the pneumococcal vaccine introduction [156, 157]. In the same pattern, vaccination in South Africa decreased the infection with penicillin-resistant strains and with trimethoprim-sulfamethoxazole-resistant strains by 67% and 56%, respectively [158]. Vaccines being developed for regularly resistant infections (such as those caused by *E.coli, S.aureus, and K.pneumoniae*, as well as *C.difficile*) reduce AMR by reducing overall selection pressure and face significant challenges [150, 151, 159].

Most of the vaccines are highly cost-effective after including the savings from reducing drug-resistance infections [160, 161]. Health care cost savings offset the cost of vaccination against Haemophilus influenzae type b conjugate vaccines (which is highly cost-effective) in all Indian states [162], while the pneumococcal vaccine was highly cost-effective in 68 of 72 developing countries [163]. For diarrheal infections, the rotavirus vaccine provided economic benefits at diverse prices, while cholera vaccination had economic benefits in certain contexts [160].

Clean and Hygiene

Even before the introduction of antibiotics, the burden of infectious diseases in the US declined largely because of improvements in water and sanitation, as Hand-washing, clean water, and excreta disposal reduce diarrheal diseases by 48%, 17%, and 36%, respectively. Many LMICs use antibiotics as a substitute for these improvements, but medications alone will not achieve the same reductions [164]. At least a 16% reduction has been observed in respiratory infections applying Hand-washing as a regular practice [165]. Hand-washing is a daily routine practice that reduces HAIs and the spread of resistant infections as confirmed by health care providers [166, 167]. Savings from averted diseases offset most investments in water, sanitation, and hygiene which otherwise requires an expensive infrastructure [168]. Water supply and sanitation interventions are non-expensive in all regions, especially hand hygiene, treated as highly cost-effective and the most affordable intervention at US$3.35 per disability-adjusted life year averted [169, 170].

Antibiotic Channel Revitalization

It is not at all surprising that the "antibiotic pipeline" is muted and needs assistance from official and unofficial sectors [81]. Earlier almost all antibiotics were discovered from soil-derived actinomycetes. This antibiotic search was efficient from the 1940s to the 1960s but slowed down for some years until the overture of linezolid in the year 2000 and daptomycin in the year 2003 [171]. Attempts have been made to produce synthetic antibiotics by alteration of existing drugs, but this has led to lesser antimicrobial activity. Also, subsequent development based on genomics and combinational chemistry, such as rational drug design and high-throughput screening, was introduced but failed to detect effective antibacterial compounds [172]. A high number of multi-channeled pharmaceutical companies rigorously developing antibiotics become scarce due to the lack of any advancement in the field along with the monetary risks.

NATIONAL POLICIES TO CONSERVE ANTIBIOTIC EFFECTIVENESS

Some countries like the United States and the United Kingdom, which belong to High-Income Countries (HICs), have enforced comprehensive national action plans. Even fewer LMICs have proved successful with such plans. So these action plans are urgently needed to be progressed in Ethiopia, South Africa, Nepal, and Vietnam.

The World Health Assembly in May 2015 passed the Global Action Plan on Antimicrobial Resistance (WHO 2015). It calls on member countries to establish national plans to address the issue of antibiotic intake and resistance (in the upcoming 2 years) [63]. The plan encompasses 5 vital objectives:

- Enhancing awareness through awareness campaigns or education.
- Strengthening available evidence via monitoring and surveillance.
- Decreasing the infection risks through preventive measures.
- Antibiotics optimization through volunteers and proper prescriptions.
- Reforming financial incentives towards new antibiotics research, albeit, preserving existing drugs.

Recommendations from Infectious Diseases Society of America's (IDSA)

Infectious Diseases Society of America (IDSA) has reported a slowdown in the development of new antibiotics because of market failure and regulatory hindrances [173].

- Reshaping of financial incentives and assistance for other joint mechanisms to address the market collapse of antibiotics.
- Latest regulatory methods to promote antimicrobial production and approval.
- Significant coordination of applicable federal agencies' efforts.
- Strengthening of antimicrobial resistance surveillance systems.
- Enhancing tasks to control and prevent AMR.
- Notable fundings in antimicrobial research.
- Significant investment in quick diagnostics R&D and incorporation into clinical practice.
- Removing unwise antibiotic use in the environment [174].

CONCLUSION

Antimicrobial resistance (AMR) is a pivotal public health issue throughout the world. While all kinds of microbial resistance are of concern, currently, resistance especially caused by bacteria is seen as most life-threatening, mainly in India. Bacteria are found in all living beings and also in soil, water, and air. With these astonishing interlinked ecosystems, the exchange of bacteria is unceasing, thus making this antibacterial resistance (ABR) problem even bigger, which is not limited to health science alone and needs a translational approach too. It requires effective collaboration among a myriad number of disciplines. The complexity of the ABR problem cannot be addressed by any individual nation independently, but more collective internationally collaborative action plans are required to tackle this ever-growing problem of drug resistance. Therefore, we are overwhelmed with the important value and presence of antibiotics as people are reliant on these drugs for the treatment of their infectious disease, and they should never be considered mere merchandise. Apart from all these, antibiotics are crucial for performing advanced surgical procedures (including organ and prosthetic transplants) successfully. Resistance mechanisms are pandemic and create an enormous clinical and economical burden on medical health care systems in the whole world. There is no so-called impeccable antibiotic, and once the most appropriate novel compounds are identified, the prescription of the antibiotic must be limited to those specified uses. If people will not change their habit of using antibiotics unnecessarily, this growing problem of resistance will never end and all futuristic drugs will have the same failing fate.

CONSENT FOR PUBLICATION

Not applicable.

CONFLICT OF INTEREST

The authors declare no conflict of interest, financial or otherwise.

ACKNOWLEDGEMENTS

S. K and Kishore acknowledge the financial assistance from the Indian council of Medical Research (ICMR). DK and SKP thank the ICMR for the senior research fellowship (SRF). MK thank the ICMR for the RA ship.

REFERENCES

[1]   Charles A Janeway J, Travers P, Walport M, Shlomchik MJ. Infectious agents and how they cause disease 2001.

[2]   Marleen MJM, Chantel WS, Carolina HP, J LFK. J LFK. Antimicrobials, chemotherapeutics or antibiotics? Sci Res Essays 2011; 6(19): 3927-9.
[http://dx.doi.org/10.5897/SRE11.406]

[3]   Antimicrobials: An Introduction — Antimicrobial Resistance Learning Site For Veterinary Students. http://amrls.cvm.msu.edu/pharmacology/antimicrobials/antimicrobials-an-introduction

[4]   Duckett S. Ernest Duchesne and the concept of fungal antibiotic therapy. Lancet 1999; 354(9195): 2068-71.
[http://dx.doi.org/10.1016/S0140-6736(99)03162-1] [PMID: 10636385]

[5]   Baldry P. The battle against bacteria: A fresh look.

[6]   Armstrong GL, Conn LA, Pinner RW. Trends in infectious disease mortality in the United States during the 20th century. JAMA 1999; 281(1): 61-6.
[http://dx.doi.org/10.1001/jama.281.1.61] [PMID: 9892452]

[7]   Aminov RI. A brief history of the antibiotic era: lessons learned and challenges for the future. Front Microbiol 2010; 1: 134.
[http://dx.doi.org/10.3389/fmicb.2010.00134] [PMID: 21687759]

[8]   Abraham EP, Chain E. An enzyme from bacteria able to destroy penicillin. Rev Infect Dis 1988; 10(4): 677-8.
[PMID: 3055168]

[9]   Davies J, Davies D. Origins and evolution of antibiotic resistance. Microbiol Mol Biol Rev 2010; 74(3): 417-33.
[http://dx.doi.org/10.1128/MMBR.00016-10] [PMID: 20805405]

[10]   Cui L, Su XZ. Discovery, mechanisms of action and combination therapy of artemisinin. Expert Rev Anti Infect Ther 2009; 7(8): 999-1013.
[http://dx.doi.org/10.1586/eri.09.68] [PMID: 19803708]

[11]   Wong RWK, Hägg U, Samaranayake L, Yuen MKZ, Seneviratne CJ, Kao R. Antimicrobial activity of Chinese medicine herbs against common bacteria in oral biofilm. A pilot study. Int J Oral Maxillofac Implants 2010; 39(6): 599-605.
[http://dx.doi.org/10.1016/j.ijom.2010.02.024] [PMID: 20418062]

[12]   Abraham EP, Chain E. An Enzyme from Bacteria able to Destroy Penicillin. Nature 1940; 146(3713): 837-7.
[http://dx.doi.org/10.1038/146837a0]

[13]   Davies J. Vicious circles: looking back on resistance plasmids. Genetics 1995; 139(4): 1465-8.
[http://dx.doi.org/10.1093/genetics/139.4.1465] [PMID: 7789752]

[14]   Helinski DR. Introduction to plasmids: a selective view of their history. In: Funnell BE, Phillips GJ, Eds. Plasmid Biology, Washington. DC, USA: ASM Press 2004; pp. 1-21.
[http://dx.doi.org/10.1128/9781555817732.ch1]

[15]   Aminov RI, Mackie RI. Evolution and ecology of antibiotic resistance genes. FEMS Microbiol Lett 2007; 271(2): 147-61.
[http://dx.doi.org/10.1111/j.1574-6968.2007.00757.x] [PMID: 17490428]

[16]   Memish ZA, Venkatesh S, Shibl AM. Impact of travel on international spread of antimicrobial resistance. Int J Antimicrob Agents 2003; 21(2): 135-42.
[http://dx.doi.org/10.1016/S0924-8579(02)00363-1] [PMID: 12615377]

[17]   Schwartz KL, Morris SK. Travel and the spread of drug-resistant bacteria. Curr Infect Dis Rep 2018; 20(9): 29.
[http://dx.doi.org/10.1007/s11908-018-0634-9] [PMID: 29959541]

[18]   Prestinaci F, Pezzotti P, Pantosti A. Antimicrobial resistance: a global multifaceted phenomenon. Pathog Glob Health 2015; 109(7): 309-18.
[http://dx.doi.org/10.1179/2047773215Y.0000000030] [PMID: 26343252]

[19]   https://www.cdc.gov/drugresistance/

[20]   https://www.who.int/news-room/fact-sheets/detail/antimicrobial-resistance

[21]   Shanmugakani RK, Srinivasan B, Glesby MJ, *et al.* Current state of the art in rapid diagnostics for antimicrobial resistance. Lab Chip 2020; 20(15): 2607-25.
[http://dx.doi.org/10.1039/D0LC00034E] [PMID: 32644060]

[22]   Gandra S, Klein EY, Pant S, Malhotra-Kumar S, Laxminarayan R. Faropenem consumption is increasing in india. Clin Infect Dis 2016; 62(8): 1050-2.
[http://dx.doi.org/10.1093/cid/ciw055] [PMID: 26908807]

[23]   Mendelson M, Røttingen J-A, Gopinathan U, *et al.* Maximising access to achieve appropriate human antimicrobial use in low-income and middle-income countries. Lancet 2016; 387(10014): 188-98.
[http://dx.doi.org/10.1016/S0140-6736(15)00547-4] [PMID: 26603919]

[24]   https://www.csis.org/analysis/us-government-and-antimicrobial-resistance

[25]   Dadgostar P. Antimicrobial resistance: implications and costs. Infect Drug Resist 2019; 12: 3903-10.
         [http://dx.doi.org/10.2147/IDR.S234610] [PMID: 31908502]

[26]   https://www.cidrap.umn.edu/news-perspective/2018/11/european-study-33000-deaths-year-res-
         stant-infections

[27]   Acharya KP, Wilson RT. Antimicrobial Resistance in Nepal. Front Med (Lausanne) 2019; 6: 105.
         [http://dx.doi.org/10.3389/fmed.2019.00105] [PMID: 31179281]

[28]   Ghenghesh KS, Rahouma A, Tawil K, Zorgani A, Franka E. Antimicrobial resistance in Libya: 1970-
         2011. Libyan J Med 2013; 8(1): 1-8.
         [http://dx.doi.org/10.3402/ljm.v8i0.20567] [PMID: 23537612]

[29]   Mustafa A. Factors leading to acquired bacterial resistance due to antibiotics. CTBM 2018; 1(1).
         [http://dx.doi.org/10.32474/CTBM.2018.01.000101]

[30]   Al-Emran HM, Eibach D, Krumkamp R, *et al.* A Multicountry Molecular Analysis of Salmonella
         enterica Serovar Typhi With Reduced Susceptibility to Ciprofloxacin in Sub-Saharan Africa. Clin
         Infect Dis 2016; 62 (Suppl. 1): S42-6.
         [http://dx.doi.org/10.1093/cid/civ788] [PMID: 26933020]

[31]   Kariuki S, Gordon MA, Feasey N, Parry CM. Antimicrobial resistance and management of invasive
         Salmonella disease. Vaccine 2015; 33 (Suppl. 3): C21-9.
         [http://dx.doi.org/10.1016/j.vaccine.2015.03.102] [PMID: 25912288]

[32]   Kumar SG, Adithan C, Harish BN, Sujatha S, Roy G, Malini A. Antimicrobial resistance in India: A
         review. J Nat Sci Biol Med 2013; 4(2): 286-91.
         [http://dx.doi.org/10.4103/0976 9668.116970] [PMID: 24082718]

[33]   https://cddep.org/publications/scoping-report-antimicrobial-resistance-india/ n.d.

[34]   Dixit A, Kumar N, Kumar S, Trigun V. Antimicrobial Resistance: Progress in the Decade since
         Emergence of New Delhi Metallo-β-Lactamase in India. Indian J Community Med 2019; 44(1): 4-8.
         [http://dx.doi.org/10.4103/ijcm.IJCM_217_18] [PMID: 30983704]

[35]   Kakkar M, Walia K, Vong S, Chatterjee P, Sharma A. Antibiotic resistance and its containment in
         India. BMJ 2017; 358: j2687.
         [http://dx.doi.org/10.1136/bmj.j2687] [PMID: 28874365]

[36]   Taneja N, Sharma M. Antimicrobial resistance in the environment: The Indian scenario. Indian J Med
         Res 2019; 149(2): 119-28.
         [http://dx.doi.org/10.4103/ijmr.IJMR_331_18] [PMID: 31219076]

[37]   Gandra S, Mojica N, Klein EY, *et al.* Trends in antibiotic resistance among major bacterial pathogens
         isolated from blood cultures tested at a large private laboratory network in India, 2008-2014. Int J
         Infect Dis 2016; 50: 75-82.
         [http://dx.doi.org/10.1016/j.ijid.2016.08.002] [PMID: 27522002]

[38]   Bonatelli ML, Oliveira LMA, Pinto TCA. Superbugs among us: who they are and what can you do to
         help win the fight? Front Young Minds 2020; 8: 5.
         [http://dx.doi.org/10.3389/frym.2020.00005]

[39]   Mulani MS, Kamble EE, Kumkar SN, Tawre MS, Pardesi KR. Emerging strategies to combat
         ESKAPE pathogens in the era of antimicrobial resistance: A review. Front Microbiol 2019; 10: 539.
         [http://dx.doi.org/10.3389/fmicb.2019.00539] [PMID: 30988669]

[40]   Magiorakos AP, Srinivasan A, Carey RB, *et al.* Multidrug-resistant, extensively drug-resistant and
         pandrug-resistant bacteria: an international expert proposal for interim standard definitions for
         acquired resistance. Clin Microbiol Infect 2012; 18(3): 268-81.
         [http://dx.doi.org/10.1111/j.1469-0691.2011.03570.x] [PMID: 21793988]

[41]   Dey S, Gaur M, Sahoo RK, *et al.* Genomic characterization of XDR Klebsiella pneumoniae ST147 co-resistant to carbapenem and colistin - The first report in India. J Glob Antimicrob Resist 2020; 22: 54-6.
[http://dx.doi.org/10.1016/j.jgar.2020.05.005] [PMID: 32470551]

[42]   Bian X, Liu X, Feng M, *et al.* Enhanced bacterial killing with colistin/sulbactam combination against carbapenem-resistant Acinetobacter baumannii. Int J Antimicrob Agents 2021; 57(2): 106271.
[http://dx.doi.org/10.1016/j.ijantimicag.2020.106271] [PMID: 33352235]

[43]   Breidenstein EBM, de la Fuente-Núñez C, Hancock REW. *Pseudomonas aeruginosa*: all roads lead to resistance. Trends Microbiol 2011; 19(8): 419-26.
[http://dx.doi.org/10.1016/j.tim.2011.04.005] [PMID: 21664819]

[44]   Mohapatra PR. Metallo-β-lactamase 1--why blame New Delhi & India? Indian J Med Res 2013; 137(1): 213-5.
[PMID: 23481076]

[45]   Viana AT, Caetano T, Covas C, Santos T, Mendo S. Environmental superbugs: The case study of Pedobacter spp. Environ Pollut 2018; 241: 1048-55.
[http://dx.doi.org/10.1016/j.envpol.2018.06.047] [PMID: 30029312]

[46]   Bandy A. Ringing bells: Morganella morganii fights for recognition. Public Health 2020; 182: 45-50.
[http://dx.doi.org/10.1016/j.puhe.2020.01.016] [PMID: 32169625]

[47]   Masi M, Pagès J-M. Structure, Function and Regulation of Outer Membrane Proteins Involved in Drug Transport in Enterobacericeae: the OmpF/C - TolC Case. Open Microbiol J 2013; 7(1): 22-33.
[http://dx.doi.org/10.2174/1874285801307010022] [PMID: 23569467]

[48]   Trott D. β-lactam resistance in gram-negative pathogens isolated from animals. Curr Pharm Des 2013; 19(2): 239-49.
[http://dx.doi.org/10.2174/138161213804070339] [PMID: 22894614]

[49]   Rubin JE, Pitout JDD. Extended-spectrum β-lactamase, carbapenemase and AmpC producing Enterobacteriaceae in companion animals. Vet Microbiol 2014; 170(1-2): 10-8.
[http://dx.doi.org/10.1016/j.vetmic.2014.01.017] [PMID: 24576841]

[50]   Brincat JP, Carosati E, Sabatini S, *et al.* Discovery of novel inhibitors of the NorA multidrug transporter of *Staphylococcus aureus*. J Med Chem 2011; 54(1): 354-65.
[http://dx.doi.org/10.1021/jm1011963] [PMID: 21141825]

[51]   Fernández-Villa D, Aguilar MR, Rojo L. Folic acid antagonists: antimicrobial and immunomodulating mechanisms and applications. Int J Mol Sci 2019; 20(20): E4996.
[http://dx.doi.org/10.3390/ijms20204996] [PMID: 31601031]

[52]   Spratt BG. Resistance to antibiotics mediated by target alterations. Science 1994; 264(5157): 388-93.
[http://dx.doi.org/10.1126/science.8153626] [PMID: 8153626]

[53]   Fleming A. Penicillin-its Discovery, Development, and Uses in the Field of Medicine and Surgery.[Harben Lectures, 1944] Lecture I. Discovery and Development of Penicillin. J R Inst Public Health 1945.

[54]   Vuckovic N, Nichter M. Changing patterns of pharmaceutical practice in the United States. Soc Sci Med 1997; 44(9): 1285-302.
[http://dx.doi.org/10.1016/S0277-9536(96)00257-2] [PMID: 9141162]

[55]   Bell BG, Schellevis F, Stobberingh E, Goossens H, Pringle M. A systematic review and meta-analysis of the effects of antibiotic consumption on antibiotic resistance. BMC Infect Dis 2014; 14(1): 13.
[http://dx.doi.org/10.1186/1471-2334-14-13] [PMID: 24405683]

[56]   Nepal G, Bhatta S. Self-medication with Antibiotics in WHO Southeast Asian Region: A Systematic Review. Cureus 2018; 10(4): e2428.
[http://dx.doi.org/10.7759/cureus.2428] [PMID: 29876150]

[57] Ateshim Y, Bereket B, Major F, *et al.* Prevalence of self-medication with antibiotics and associated factors in the community of Asmara, Eritrea: a descriptive cross sectional survey. BMC Public Health 2019; 19(1): 726.
[http://dx.doi.org/10.1186/s12889-019-7020-x] [PMID: 31182071]

[58] D'Costa VM, King CE, Kalan L, *et al.* Antibiotic resistance is ancient. Nature 2011; 477(7365): 457-61.
[http://dx.doi.org/10.1038/nature10388] [PMID: 21881561]

[59] Holmes AH, Moore LSP, Sundsfjord A, *et al.* Understanding the mechanisms and drivers of antimicrobial resistance. Lancet 2016; 387(10014): 176-87.
[http://dx.doi.org/10.1016/S0140-6736(15)00473-0] [PMID: 26603922]

[60] Chang Q, Wang W, Regev-Yochay G, Lipsitch M, Hanage WP. Antibiotics in agriculture and the risk to human health: how worried should we be? Evol Appl 2015; 8(3): 240-7.
[http://dx.doi.org/10.1111/eva.12185] [PMID: 25861382]

[61] Pruden A, Larsson DGJ, Amézquita A, *et al.* Management options for reducing the release of antibiotics and antibiotic resistance genes to the environment. Environ Health Perspect 2013; 121(8): 878-85.
[http://dx.doi.org/10.1289/ehp.1206446] [PMID: 23735422]

[62] Martinez JL. Environmental pollution by antibiotics and by antibiotic resistance determinants. Environ Pollut 2009; 157(11): 2893-902.
[http://dx.doi.org/10.1016/j.envpol.2009.05.051] [PMID: 19560847]

[63] Miller-Petrie M, Pant S, Laxminarayan R. Drug-Resistant Infections.Major Infectious Diseases. 3rd ed., Washington, DC: The International Bank for Reconstruction and Development / The World Bank 2017.
[http://dx.doi.org/10.1596/978-1-4648-0524-0_ch18]

[64] Du H, Chen L, Tang Y-W, Kreiswirth BN. Emergence of the mcr-1 colistin resistance gene in carbapenem-resistant Enterobacteriaceae. Lancet Infect Dis 2016; 16(3): 287-8.
[http://dx.doi.org/10.1016/S1473-3099(16)00056-6] [PMID: 26842776]

[65] Johnson AP, Woodford N. Global spread of antibiotic resistance: the example of New Delhi metallo-β-lactamase (NDM)-mediated carbapenem resistance. J Med Microbiol 2013; 62(Pt 4): 499-513.
[http://dx.doi.org/10.1099/jmm.0.052555-0] [PMID: 23329317]

[66] Hargreaves S, Lönnroth K, Nellums LB, *et al.* Multidrug-resistant tuberculosis and migration to Europe. Clin Microbiol Infect 2017; 23(3): 141-6.
[http://dx.doi.org/10.1016/j.cmi.2016.09.009] [PMID: 27665703]

[67] van Hecke O, Lee JJ, O'Sullivan JW. Antimicrobial resistance among migrants in Europe. Lancet Infect Dis 2018; 18(9): 944.
[http://dx.doi.org/10.1016/S1473-3099(18)30468-7] [PMID: 30152355]

[68] MacPherson DW, Gushulak BD, Baine WB, *et al.* Population mobility, globalization, and antimicrobial drug resistance. Emerg Infect Dis 2009; 15(11): 1727-32.
[http://dx.doi.org/10.3201/eid1511.090419] [PMID: 19891858]

[69] Allcock S, Young EH, Holmes M, *et al.* Antimicrobial resistance in human populations: challenges and opportunities. Glob Health Epidemiol Genom 2017; 2: e4.
[http://dx.doi.org/10.1017/gheg.2017.4] [PMID: 29276617]

[70] Bruinsma N, Hutchinson JM, van den Bogaard AE, Giamarellou H, Degener J, Stobberingh EE. Influence of population density on antibiotic resistance. J Antimicrob Chemother 2003; 51(2): 385-90.
[http://dx.doi.org/10.1093/jac/dkg072] [PMID: 12562707]

[71] Sattar SA, Tetro J, Springthorpe VS. Impact of changing societal trends on the spread of infections in American and Canadian homes. Am J Infect Control 1999; 27(6): S4-S21.
[http://dx.doi.org/10.1016/S0196-6553(99)70037-4] [PMID: 10586141]

[72]   Karkman A, Pärnänen K, Larsson DGJ. Fecal pollution can explain antibiotic resistance gene abundances in anthropogenically impacted environments. Nat Commun 2019; 10(1): 80.
[http://dx.doi.org/10.1038/s41467-018-07992-3] [PMID: 30622259]

[73]   MacFadden DR, McGough SF, Fisman D, Santillana M, Brownstein JS. Antibiotic resistance increases with local temperature. Nat Clim Chang 2018; 8(6): 510-4.
[http://dx.doi.org/10.1038/s41558-018-0161-6] [PMID: 30369964]

[74]   De Silva PM, Chong P, Fernando DM, Westmacott G, Kumar A. Effect of Incubation Temperature on Antibiotic Resistance and Virulence Factors of Acinetobacter baumannii ATCC 17978. Antimicrob Agents Chemother 2017; 62(1): e01514-17.
[http://dx.doi.org/10.1128/AAC.01514-17] [PMID: 29061747]

[75]   Rodríguez-Verdugo A, Lozano-Huntelman N, Cruz-Loya M, Savage V, Yeh P. Compounding effects of climate warming and antibiotic resistance. iScience 2020; 23(4): 101024.
[http://dx.doi.org/10.1016/j.isci.2020.101024] [PMID: 32299057]

[76]   Klein EY, Makowsky M, Orlando M, Hatna E, Braykov NP, Laxminarayan R. Influence of provider and urgent care density across different socioeconomic strata on outpatient antibiotic prescribing in the USA. J Antimicrob Chemother 2015; 70(5): 1580-7.
[http://dx.doi.org/10.1093/jac/dku563] [PMID: 25604743]

[77]   Zhang Y, Lee BY, Donohue JM. Ambulatory antibiotic use and prescription drug coverage in older adults. Arch Intern Med 2010; 170(15): 1308-14.
[http://dx.doi.org/10.1001/archinternmed.2010.235] [PMID: 20696953]

[78]   Dosh SA, Hickner JM, Mainous AG III, Ebell MH. Predictors of antibiotic prescribing for nonspecific upper respiratory infections, acute bronchitis, and acute sinusitis. An UPRNet study. J Fam Pract 2000; 49(5): 407-14.
[PMID: 10836770]

[79]   Linder JA, Doctor JN, Friedberg MW, *et al.* Time of day and the decision to prescribe antibiotics. JAMA Intern Med 2014; 174(12): 2029-31.
[http://dx.doi.org/10.1001/jamainternmed.2014.5225] [PMID: 25286067]

[80]   Sun L, Klein EY, Laxminarayan R. Seasonality and temporal correlation between community antibiotic use and resistance in the United States. Clin Infect Dis 2012; 55(5): 687-94.
[http://dx.doi.org/10.1093/cid/cis509] [PMID: 22752512]

[81]   Woon S-A, Fisher D. Antimicrobial agents - optimising the ecological balance. BMC Med 2016; 14(1): 114.
[http://dx.doi.org/10.1186/s12916-016-0661-z] [PMID: 27495926]

[82]   Liu Y-Y, Wang Y, Walsh TR, *et al.* Emergence of plasmid-mediated colistin resistance mechanism MCR-1 in animals and human beings in China: a microbiological and molecular biological study. Lancet Infect Dis 2016; 16(2): 161-8.
[http://dx.doi.org/10.1016/S1473-3099(15)00424-7] [PMID: 26603172]

[83]   Simjee S, McDermott P, Trott DJ, Chuanchuen R. Present and future surveillance of antimicrobial resistance in animals: principles and practices. Microbiol Spectr 2018; 6(4): 6.4.06.
[http://dx.doi.org/10.1128/microbiolspec.ARBA-0028-2017] [PMID: 30003869]

[84]   Anjum MF, Zankari E, Hasman H. Molecular methods for detection of antimicrobial resistance. Microbiol Spectr 2017; 5(6): 5.6.02.
[http://dx.doi.org/10.1128/microbiolspec.ARBA-0011-2017] [PMID: 29219107]

[85]   Feucherolles M, Cauchie H-M, Penny C. MALDI-TOF Mass Spectrometry and Specific Biomarkers: Potential New Key for Swift Identification of Antimicrobial Resistance in Foodborne Pathogens. Microorganisms 2019; 7(12): E593.
[http://dx.doi.org/10.3390/microorganisms7120593] [PMID: 31766422]

[86]   Banerji A, Jahne M, Herrmann M, Brinkman N, Keely S. Bringing community ecology to bear on the

issue of antimicrobial resistance. Front Microbiol 2019; 10: 2626.
[http://dx.doi.org/10.3389/fmicb.2019.02626] [PMID: 31803161]

[87]   Boolchandani M, D'Souza AW, Dantas G. Sequencing-based methods and resources to study antimicrobial resistance. Nat Rev Genet 2019; 20(6): 356-70.
[http://dx.doi.org/10.1038/s41576-019-0108-4] [PMID: 30886350]

[88]   Kim J, Greenberg DE, Pifer R, *et al.* VAMPr: VAriant Mapping and Prediction of antibiotic resistance *via* explainable features and machine learning. PLOS Comput Biol 2020; 16(1): e1007511.
[http://dx.doi.org/10.1371/journal.pcbi.1007511] [PMID: 31929521]

[89]   Bennani H, Mateus A, Mays N, Eastmure E, Stärk KDC, Häsler B. Overview of evidence of antimicrobial use and antimicrobial resistance in the food chain. Antibiotics (Basel) 2020; 9(2): E49.
[http://dx.doi.org/10.3390/antibiotics9020049] [PMID: 32013023]

[90]   Mack I, Sharland M, Berkley JA, Klein N, Malhotra-Kumar S, Bielicki J. Antimicrobial resistance following azithromycin mass drug administration: potential surveillance strategies to assess public health impact. Clin Infect Dis 2020; 70(7): 1501-8.
[http://dx.doi.org/10.1093/cid/ciz893] [PMID: 31633161]

[91]   Pezzani MD, Mazzaferri F, Compri M, *et al.* Linking antimicrobial resistance surveillance to antibiotic policy in healthcare settings: the COMBACTE-Magnet EPI-Net COACH project. J Antimicrob Chemother 2020; 75 (Suppl. 2): ii2-ii19.
[http://dx.doi.org/10.1093/jac/dkaa425] [PMID: 33280049]

[92]   Mercer DK, Torres MDT, Duay SS, *et al.* Antimicrobial susceptibility testing of antimicrobial peptides to better predict efficacy. Front Cell Infect Microbiol 2020; 10: 326.
[http://dx.doi.org/10.3389/fcimb.2020.00326] [PMID: 32733816]

[93]   Joo SH. Lipid A as a drug target and therapeutic molecule. Biomol Ther (Seoul) 2015; 23(6): 510-6.
[http://dx.doi.org/10.4062/biomolther.2015.117] [PMID: 26535075]

[94]   Raetz CRH, Reynolds CM, Trent MS, Bishop RE. Lipid A modification systems in gram-negative bacteria. Annu Rev Biochem 2007; 76(1): 295-329.
[http://dx.doi.org/10.1146/annurev.biochem.76.010307.145803] [PMID: 17362200]

[95]   Anderson MS, Robertson AD, Macher I, Raetz CR. Biosynthesis of lipid A in Escherichia coli: identification of UDP-3-O-[(R)-3-hydroxymyristoyl]-alpha-D-glucosamine as a precursor of UDP-N2,O3-bis[(R)-3-hydroxymyristoyl]-alpha-D-glucosamine. Biochemistry 1988; 27(6): 1908-17.
[http://dx.doi.org/10.1021/bi00406a017] [PMID: 3288280]

[96]   Bulawa CE, Raetz CR. The biosynthesis of gram-negative endotoxin. Identification and function of UDP-2,3-diacylglucosamine in Escherichia coli. J Biol Chem 1984; 259(8): 4846-51.
[http://dx.doi.org/10.1016/S0021-9258(17)42923-1] [PMID: 6370994]

[97]   Anderson MS, Bulawa CE, Raetz CR. The biosynthesis of gram-negative endotoxin. Formation of lipid A precursors from UDP-GlcNAc in extracts of Escherichia coli. J Biol Chem 1985; 260(29): 15536-41.
[http://dx.doi.org/10.1016/S0021-9258(17)36289-0] [PMID: 3905795]

[98]   Raetz CRH, Guan Z, Ingram BO, *et al.* Discovery of new biosynthetic pathways: the lipid A story. J Lipid Res 2009; 50 (Suppl.): S103-8.
[http://dx.doi.org/10.1194/jlr.R800060-JLR200] [PMID: 18974037]

[99]   Clementz T, Zhou Z, Raetz CR. Function of the Escherichia coli msbB gene, a multicopy suppressor of htrB knockouts, in the acylation of lipid A. Acylation by MsbB follows laurate incorporation by HtrB. J Biol Chem 1997; 272(16): 10353-60.
[http://dx.doi.org/10.1074/jbc.272.16.10353] [PMID: 9099672]

[100] Jackman JE, Raetz CR, Fierke CA. UDP-3-O-(R-3-hydroxymyristoyl)-N-acetylglucosamine deacetylase of Escherichia coli is a zinc metalloenzyme. Biochemistry 1999; 38(6): 1902-11.
[http://dx.doi.org/10.1021/bi982339s] [PMID: 10026271]

[101] Zhou P, Barb AW. Mechanism and inhibition of LpxC: an essential zinc-dependent deacetylase of bacterial lipid A synthesis. Curr Pharm Biotechnol 2008; 9(1): 9-15.

[102] Barb AW, Zhou P. Mechanism and inhibition of LpxC: an essential zinc-dependent deacetylase of bacterial lipid A synthesis. Curr Pharm Biotechnol 2008; 9(1): 9-15.
[http://dx.doi.org/10.2174/138920108783497668] [PMID: 18289052]

[103] Barb AW, Jiang L, Raetz CRH, Zhou P. Structure of the deacetylase LpxC bound to the antibiotic CHIR-090: Time-dependent inhibition and specificity in ligand binding. Proc Natl Acad Sci USA 2007; 104(47): 18433-8.
[http://dx.doi.org/10.1073/pnas.0709412104] [PMID: 18025458]

[104] Zhang G, Meredith TC, Kahne D. On the essentiality of lipopolysaccharide to Gram-negative bacteria. Curr Opin Microbiol 2013; 16(6): 779-85.
[http://dx.doi.org/10.1016/j.mib.2013.09.007] [PMID: 24148302]

[105] Delucia AM, Six DA, Caughlan RE, *et al.* Lipopolysaccharide (LPS) inner-core phosphates are required for complete LPS synthesis and transport to the outer membrane in *Pseudomonas aeruginosa* PAO1. MBio 2011; 2(4): e00142-11.
[http://dx.doi.org/10.1128/mBio.00142-11] [PMID: 21810964]

[106] Onishi HR, Pelak BA, Gerckens LS, *et al.* Antibacterial agents that inhibit lipid A biosynthesis. Science 1996; 274(5289): 980-2.
[http://dx.doi.org/10.1126/science.274.5289.980] [PMID: 8875939]

[107] McClerren AL, Endsley S, Bowman JL, *et al.* A slow, tight-binding inhibitor of the zinc-dependent deacetylase LpxC of lipid A biosynthesis with antibiotic activity comparable to ciprofloxacin. Biochemistry 2005; 44(50): 16574-83.
[http://dx.doi.org/10.1021/bi0518186] [PMID: 16342948]

[108] Liang X, Lee C-J, Zhao J, Toone EJ, Zhou P. Synthesis, structure, and antibiotic activity of aryl-substituted LpxC inhibitors. J Med Chem 2013; 56(17): 6954-66.
[http://dx.doi.org/10.1021/jm4007774] [PMID: 23914798]

[109] Payne DJ, Gwynn MN, Holmes DJ, Pompliano DL. Drugs for bad bugs: confronting the challenges of antibacterial discovery. Nat Rev Drug Discov 2007; 6(1): 29-40.
[http://dx.doi.org/10.1038/nrd2201] [PMID: 17159923]

[110] Clatworthy AE, Pierson E, Hung DT. Targeting virulence: a new paradigm for antimicrobial therapy. Nat Chem Biol 2007; 3(9): 541-8.
[http://dx.doi.org/10.1038/nchembio.2007.24] [PMID: 17710100]

[111] Negrea A, Bjur E, Ygberg SE, Elofsson M, Wolf-Watz H, Rhen M. Salicylidene acylhydrazides that affect type III protein secretion in Salmonella enterica serovar typhimurium. Antimicrob Agents Chemother 2007; 51(8): 2867-76.
[http://dx.doi.org/10.1128/AAC.00223-07] [PMID: 17548496]

[112] Rasko DA, Moreira CG, Li R, *et al.* Targeting QseC signaling and virulence for antibiotic development. Science 2008; 321(5892): 1078-80.
[http://dx.doi.org/10.1126/science.1160354] [PMID: 18719281]

[113] Liu C-I, Liu GY, Song Y, *et al.* A cholesterol biosynthesis inhibitor blocks *Staphylococcus aureus* virulence. Science 2008; 319(5868): 1391-4.
[http://dx.doi.org/10.1126/science.1153018] [PMID: 18276850]

[114] Lock RL, Harry EJ. Cell-division inhibitors: new insights for future antibiotics. Nat Rev Drug Discov 2008; 7(4): 324-38.
[http://dx.doi.org/10.1038/nrd2510] [PMID: 18323848]

[115] Gotoh Y, Eguchi Y, Watanabe T, Okamoto S, Doi A, Utsumi R. Two-component signal transduction as potential drug targets in pathogenic bacteria. Curr Opin Microbiol 2010; 13(2): 232-9.
[http://dx.doi.org/10.1016/j.mib.2010.01.008] [PMID: 20138000]

[116] Njoroge J, Sperandio V. Jamming bacterial communication: new approaches for the treatment of infectious diseases. EMBO Mol Med 2009; 1(4): 201-10.
[http://dx.doi.org/10.1002/emmm.200900032] [PMID: 20049722]

[117] Su Z, Honek JF. Emerging bacterial enzyme targets. Curr Opin Investig Drugs 2007; 8(2): 140-9.
[PMID: 17328230]

[118] Schimmel P, Tao J, Hill J. Aminoacyl tRNA synthetases as targets for new anti-infectives. FASEB J 1998; 12(15): 1599-609.
[http://dx.doi.org/10.1096/fasebj.12.15.1599] [PMID: 9837850]

[119] Diacon AH, Pym A, Grobusch M, *et al.* The diarylquinoline TMC207 for multidrug-resistant tuberculosis. N Engl J Med 2009; 360(23): 2397-405.
[http://dx.doi.org/10.1056/NEJMoa0808427] [PMID: 19494215]

[120] Bush K, Macielag MJ. New β-lactam antibiotics and β-lactamase inhibitors. Expert Opin Ther Pat 2010; 20(10): 1277-93.
[http://dx.doi.org/10.1517/13543776.2010.515588] [PMID: 20839927]

[121] Lomovskaya O, Bostian KA. Practical applications and feasibility of efflux pump inhibitors in the clinic--a vision for applied use. Biochem Pharmacol 2006; 71(7): 910-8.
[http://dx.doi.org/10.1016/j.bcp.2005.12.008] [PMID: 16427026]

[122] Kohanski MA, DePristo MA, Collins JJ. Sublethal antibiotic treatment leads to multidrug resistance *via* radical-induced mutagenesis. Mol Cell 2010; 37(3): 311-20.
[http://dx.doi.org/10.1016/j.molcel.2010.01.003] [PMID: 20159551]

[123] Lu TK, Collins JJ. Engineered bacteriophage targeting gene networks as adjuvants for antibiotic therapy. Proc Natl Acad Sci USA 2009; 106(12): 4629-34.
[http://dx.doi.org/10.1073/pnas.0800442106] [PMID: 19255432]

[124] Mendelson M, Morris AM, Thursky K, Pulcini C. How to start an antimicrobial stewardship programme in a hospital. Clin Microbiol Infect 2020; 26(4): 447-53.
[http://dx.doi.org/10.1016/j.cmi.2019.08.007] [PMID: 31445209]

[125] Briceland LL, Nightingale CH, Quintiliani R, Cooper BW, Smith KS. Antibiotic streamlining from combination therapy to monotherapy utilizing an interdisciplinary approach. Arch Intern Med 1988; 148(9): 2019-22.
[http://dx.doi.org/10.1001/archinte.1988.00380090091022] [PMID: 3415406]

[126] Fraser GL, Stogsdill P, Dickens JD Jr, Wennberg DE, Smith RP Jr, Prato BS. Antibiotic optimization. An evaluation of patient safety and economic outcomes. Arch Intern Med 1997; 157(15): 1689-94.
[http://dx.doi.org/10.1001/archinte.1997.00440360105012] [PMID: 9250230]

[127] Fraser G, Stogsdill P, Owens RC, Ambrose PG. Antibiotic optimization: Concepts and strategies in clinical practice.

[128] Owens RC Jr, Fraser GL, Stogsdill P. Antimicrobial stewardship programs as a means to optimize antimicrobial use. Pharmacotherapy 2004; 24(7): 896-908.
[http://dx.doi.org/10.1592/phco.24.9.896.36101] [PMID: 15303453]

[129] Glowacki RC, Schwartz DN, Itokazu GS, Wisniewski MF, Kieszkowski P, Weinstein RA. Antibiotic combinations with redundant antimicrobial spectra: clinical epidemiology and pilot intervention of computer-assisted surveillance. Clin Infect Dis 2003; 37(1): 59-64.
[http://dx.doi.org/10.1086/376623] [PMID: 12830409]

[130] Maki G, Smith I, Paulin S, *et al.* Feasibility Study of the World Health Organization Health Care Facility-Based Antimicrobial Stewardship Toolkit for Low- and Middle-Income Countries. Antibiotics (Basel) 2020; 9(9): E556.
[http://dx.doi.org/10.3390/antibiotics9090556] [PMID: 32872440]

[131] Morgan DJ, Okeke IN, Laxminarayan R, Perencevich EN, Weisenberg S. Non-prescription

antimicrobial use worldwide: a systematic review. Lancet Infect Dis 2011; 11(9): 692-701.
[http://dx.doi.org/10.1016/S1473-3099(11)70054-8] [PMID: 21659004]

[132]   Bartoloni A, Cutts F, Leoni S, *et al.* Patterns of antimicrobial use and antimicrobial resistance among healthy children in Bolivia. Trop Med Int Health 1998; 3(2): 116-23.
[http://dx.doi.org/10.1046/j.1365-3156.1998.00201.x] [PMID: 9537273]

[133]   Thamlikitkul V. Antibiotic dispensing by drug store personnel in Bangkok, Thailand. J Antimicrob Chemother 1988; 21(1): 125-31.
[http://dx.doi.org/10.1093/jac/21.1.125] [PMID: 3356619]

[134]   Awad A, Eltayeb I, Matowe L, Thalib L. Self-medication with antibiotics and antimalarials in the community of Khartoum State, Sudan. J Pharm Pharm Sci 2005; 8(2): 326-31.
[PMID: 16124943]

[135]   Land T. Combating counterfeit drugs. Nature 1992; 355(6357): 192.
[http://dx.doi.org/10.1038/355192a0] [PMID: 1731208]

[136]   Taylor RB, Shakoor O, Behrens RH. Drug quality, a contributor to drug resistance? Lancet 1995; 346(8967): 122.
[http://dx.doi.org/10.1016/S0140-6736(95)92145-1] [PMID: 7603195]

[137]   Okeke IN, Lamikanra A. Quality and bioavailability of tetracycline capsules in a Nigerian semi-urban community. Int J Antimicrob Agents 1995; 5(4): 245-50.
[http://dx.doi.org/10.1016/0924-8579(94)00064-2] [PMID: 18611675]

[138]   Park S, Soumerai SB, Adams AS, Finkelstein JA, Jang S, Ross-Degnan D. Antibiotic use following a Korean national policy to prohibit medication dispensing by physicians. Health Policy Plan 2005; 20(5): 302-9.
[http://dx.doi.org/10.1093/heapol/czi033] [PMID: 16000369]

[139]   Bavestrello L, Cabello A, Casanova D. Impact of regulatory measures in the trends of community consumption of antibiotics in Chile. Rev Med Chil 2002; 130(11): 1265-72.
[PMID: 12587509]

[140]   Stokstad ELR, Jukes TH. Further observations on the "animal protein factor. Exp Biol Med (Maywood) 1950; 73(3): 523-8.
[http://dx.doi.org/10.3181/00379727-73-17731]

[141]   Stahly TS, Cromwell GL, Monegue HJ. Effects of the dietary inclusion of copper and(or) antibiotics on the performance of weanling pigs. J Anim Sci 1980; 51(6): 1347-51.
[http://dx.doi.org/10.2527/jas1981.5161347x] [PMID: 6782067]

[142]   Alexander TW, Yanke LJ, Topp E, *et al.* Effect of subtherapeutic administration of antibiotics on the prevalence of antibiotic-resistant Escherichia coli bacteria in feedlot cattle. Appl Environ Microbiol 2008; 74(14): 4405-16.
[http://dx.doi.org/10.1128/AEM.00489-08] [PMID: 18502931]

[143]   Cho I, Yamanishi S, Cox L, *et al.* Antibiotics in early life alter the murine colonic microbiome and adiposity. Nature 2012; 488(7413): 621-6.
[http://dx.doi.org/10.1038/nature11400] [PMID: 22914093]

[144]   Maron DF, Smith TJS, Nachman KE. Restrictions on antimicrobial use in food animal production: an international regulatory and economic survey. Global Health 2013; 9(1): 48.
[http://dx.doi.org/10.1186/1744 8603 9 48] [PMID: 24131666]

[145]   https://www.medscape.com/viewarticle/845820 n.d.

[146]   Goodridge LD, Bisha B. Phage-based biocontrol strategies to reduce foodborne pathogens in foods. Bacteriophage 2011; 1(3): 130-7.
[http://dx.doi.org/10.4161/bact.1.3.17629] [PMID: 22164346]

[147]   Balogh B, Jones JB, Iriarte FB, Momol MT. Phage therapy for plant disease control. Curr Pharm

Biotechnol 2010; 11(1): 48-57.
[http://dx.doi.org/10.2174/138920110790725302] [PMID: 20214607]

[148] Allen HK, Trachsel J, Looft T, Casey TA. Finding alternatives to antibiotics. Ann N Y Acad Sci 2014; 1323(1): 91-100.
[http://dx.doi.org/10.1111/nyas.12468] [PMID: 24953233]

[149] Kadouri DE, To K, Shanks RMQ, Doi Y. Predatory bacteria: a potential ally against multidrug-resistant Gram-negative pathogens. PLoS One 2013; 8(5): e63397.
[http://dx.doi.org/10.1371/journal.pone.0063397] [PMID: 23650563]

[150] Kwong JC, Maaten S, Upshur REG, Patrick DM, Marra F. The effect of universal influenza immunization on antibiotic prescriptions: an ecological study. Clin Infect Dis 2009; 49(5): 750-6.
[http://dx.doi.org/10.1086/605087] [PMID: 19624280]

[151] Polgreen PM, Yang M, Laxminarayan R, Cavanaugh JE. Respiratory fluoroquinolone use and influenza. Infect Control Hosp Epidemiol 2011; 32(7): 706-9.
[http://dx.doi.org/10.1086/660859] [PMID: 21666403]

[152] McCullers JA. The co-pathogenesis of influenza viruses with bacteria in the lung. Nat Rev Microbiol 2014; 12(4): 252-62.
[http://dx.doi.org/10.1038/nrmicro3231] [PMID: 24590244]

[153] Falsey AR, Becker KL, Swinburne AJ, *et al.* Bacterial complications of respiratory tract viral illness: a comprehensive evaluation. J Infect Dis 2013; 208(3): 432-41.
[http://dx.doi.org/10.1093/infdis/jit190] [PMID: 23661797]

[154] Okeke IN. Cholera vaccine will reduce antibiotic use. Science 2009; 325(5941): 674.
[http://dx.doi.org/10.1126/science.325_674b] [PMID: 19661401]

[155] Ganguly NK, Arora NK, Chandy SJ, *et al.* Rationalizing antibiotic use to limit antibiotic resistance in India. Indian J Med Res 2011; 134: 281-94.
[PMID: 21985810]

[156] Grijalva CG, Nuorti JP, Arbogast PG, Martin SW, Edwards KM, Griffin MR. Decline in pneumonia admissions after routine childhood immunisation with pneumococcal conjugate vaccine in the USA: a time-series analysis. Lancet 2007; 369(9568): 1179-86.
[http://dx.doi.org/10.1016/S0140-6736(07)60564-9] [PMID: 17416262]

[157] Kyaw MH, Lynfield R, Schaffner W, *et al.* Effect of introduction of the pneumococcal conjugate vaccine on drug-resistant Streptococcus pneumoniae. N Engl J Med 2006; 354(14): 1455-63.
[http://dx.doi.org/10.1056/NEJMoa051642] [PMID: 16598044]

[158] Klugman KP, Madhi SA, Huebner RE, Kohberger R, Mbelle N, Pierce N. A trial of a 9-valent pneumococcal conjugate vaccine in children with and those without HIV infection. N Engl J Med 2003; 349(14): 1341-8.
[http://dx.doi.org/10.1056/NEJMoa035060] [PMID: 14523142]

[159] https://cddep.org/publications/state_worlds_antibiotics_2015/ n.d.

[160] Rheingans R, Amaya M, Anderson JD, Chakraborty P, Atem J. Systematic review of the economic value of diarrheal vaccines. Hum Vaccin Immunother 2014; 10(6): 1582-94.
[http://dx.doi.org/10.4161/hv.29352] [PMID: 24861846]

[161] https://www.who.int/immunization/sowvi/en/

[162] Clark AD, Griffiths UK, Abbas SS, *et al.* Impact and cost-effectiveness of Haemophilus influenzae type b conjugate vaccination in India. J Pediatr 2013; 163(1) (Suppl.): S60-72.
[http://dx.doi.org/10.1016/j.jpeds.2013.03.032] [PMID: 23773596]

[163] Sinha A, Levine O, Knoll MD, Muhib F, Lieu TA. Cost-effectiveness of pneumococcal conjugate vaccination in the prevention of child mortality: an international economic analysis. Lancet 2007; 369(9559): 389-96.

[http://dx.doi.org/10.1016/S0140-6736(07)60195-0] [PMID: 17276779]

[164] Cairncross S, Hunt C, Boisson S, *et al.* Water, sanitation and hygiene for the prevention of diarrhoea. Int J Epidemiol 2010; 39 (Suppl. 1): i193-205.
[http://dx.doi.org/10.1093/ije/dyq035] [PMID: 20348121]

[165] Rabie T, Curtis V. Handwashing and risk of respiratory infections: a quantitative systematic review. Trop Med Int Health 2006; 11(3): 258-67.
[http://dx.doi.org/10.1111/j.1365-3156.2006.01568.x] [PMID: 16553905]

[166] Allegranzi B, Pittet D. Role of hand hygiene in healthcare-associated infection prevention. J Hosp Infect 2009; 73(4): 305-15.
[http://dx.doi.org/10.1016/j.jhin.2009.04.019] [PMID: 19720430]

[167] De Angelis G, Cataldo MA, De Waure C, *et al.* Infection control and prevention measures to reduce the spread of vancomycin-resistant enterococci in hospitalized patients: a systematic review and meta-analysis. J Antimicrob Chemother 2014; 69(5): 1185-92.
[http://dx.doi.org/10.1093/jac/dkt525] [PMID: 24458513]

[168] Public Health and the Environment Water, Sanitation and Hygiene.

[169] Jamison DT, Breman JG, Measham AR, Alleyne G, Claeson M, Evans DB, Eds. Disease control priorities in developing countries. 2nd ed., Washington, DC: World Bank 2006.

[170] Hutton G, Haller L, Bartram J. Global cost-benefit analysis of water supply and sanitation interventions. J Water Health 2007; 5(4): 481-502.
[http://dx.doi.org/10.2166/wh.2007.009] [PMID: 17878562]

[171] Boucher HW, Talbot GH, Benjamin DK Jr, *et al.* 10 x '20 Progress--development of new drugs active against gram-negative bacilli: an update from the Infectious Diseases Society of America. Clin Infect Dis 2013; 56(12): 1685-94.
[http://dx.doi.org/10.1093/cid/cit152] [PMID: 23599308]

[172] Lewis K. Platforms for antibiotic discovery. Nat Rev Drug Discov 2013; 12(5): 371-87.
[http://dx.doi.org/10.1038/nrd3975] [PMID: 23629505]

[173] http://drive-ab.eu/news/idsa-releases-new-antibiotic-stewardship-guidelines-with-focus-on-practical-advice-for-implementation/ n.d.

[174] Spellberg B, Blaser M, Guidos RJ, *et al.* Combating antimicrobial resistance: policy recommendations to save lives. Clin Infect Dis 2011; 52 (Suppl. 5): S397-428.
[http://dx.doi.org/10.1093/cid/cir153] [PMID: 21474585]

CHAPTER 10

Drug Discovery for MDR

Jyoti Yadav[1], Nagendra Singh[2], Anupam Jyoti[3], Vijay Kumar Srivastava[1], Vinay Sharma[1] and Sanket Kaushik[1,*]

[1] *Amity Institute of Biotechnology, Amity University Rajasthan, Jaipur-303002, India*

[2] *School of Biotechnology, Gautam Buddha University, Greater Noida, India*

[3] *Department of Biotechnology, University Institute of Biotechnology, Chandigarh University, Chandigarh, India*

Abstract: Infections caused by MDR (Multi-drug resistant) strains are increasing with time due to the selection pressure posed by the use of antibiotics. The mechanisms that confer antibiotic resistance to bacteria are gene mutation, change in cell envelop, over expression of efflux pumps and biofilm formation. Drug development for MDR has become one of the major challenges globally. MDR infections associated with health care facilities are difficult to treat due to the limited therapeutic approaches or even no treatment options. Therefore, there is an emergency to develop new therapeutic approaches against MDR pathogens. It is possible to identify proteins that are responsible for the survival of pathogenic MDR bacteria for the purpose of drug discovery. Rational-structure based drug design is an inventive process of finding new drug targets, which relies on the knowledge of three-dimensional structure of biological targets. The three-dimension structure is obtained by high throughput techniques such as X-ray diffraction (XRD), Nuclear Magnetic Resonance (NMR) and Cryo-electron microscopy (Cryo- EM). Structure biology plays an important role in the characterization of new therapeutic targets and assessment of drug targets. Computational methods boost drug development and discovery process against MDR pathogens and analyse efficient therapies.

Keywords: Antibiotic resistance, Cryo-EM, Drug discovery, Multidrug resistance, NMR, Rational structure based drug design, Structure biology, X-ray diffraction.

INTRODUCTION

Over the past decade, emergence of antimicrobial resistance in pathogenic bacteria has become a major public health concern all over the world. Treatment

* **Corresponding author Sanket Kaushik:** Amity Institute of Biotechnology, Amity University Rajasthan, Jaipur-303002, India; E-mail: sanketkaushik@gmail.com

of several bacterial infections has become increasingly difficult due to the emergence of multidrug resistant strains [1 - 3]. Antibiotics resistance may arise as a result of mutations in the gene, changes in cell envelop, over-expression of efflux pumps, biofilm formation, *etc.* [4, 5]. Multi-drug resistance to different antibiotics develops due to inappropriate use of antibiotics, poor infection prevention and insufficient conditions of sanity [4, 6, 7]. There are several clinical isolates that have developed antibiotic resistant and are more commonly found in hospital environments, such as methicillin resistant *Staphylococcus aureus* (MRSA), vancomycin resistant *Enterococci* (VRE) and the members of the *Enterobacteriaceae* family [8, 9]. Drug development against such multi-drug resistant bacterial strains has become one of the major challenges for medicinal industries [10]. In this regard, it is possible to target essential proteins for the survival of the bacteria for the purpose of drug discovery [11, 12]. Rational structural-based drug design is the process of finding small molecule inhibitors based on the knowledge of three-dimensional structure of biological target proteins [13]. The three-dimensional structures of the targets are obtained by high throughput techniques such as X-ray crystallography, nuclear magnetic resonance (NMR), spectroscopy or cryo-electron microscopy (cryo-EM) [14, 15]. The three-dimensional structure of the target molecule is used to predict candidate drug molecules that selectively and tightly interact with binding sites of the protein or enzyme of the pathogenic microbe. The small molecule inhibitors are chosen as lead molecules against the target [16]. Dorzolamide, saquinavir, zanamivir and imatinib which target carbonic anhydrase, HIV protease, neuraminidase and BCR-ABL respectively, are some of the examples of successful cases of structural-based drug design [16].

EMERGENCE OF MULTIDRUG RESISTANCE IN BACTERIA

Multi-drug resistance associated with unselective use of prolonged exposure to antibiotics led to excess morbidity, mortality and high cost in clinical settings. It also increased the prevalence of pathogenic multi-drug resistant bacteria globally [17]. It has been noted that over the last few decade plasmid-borne resistance genes and cross resistance are the major factors that facilitates the process of resistance in bacteria [18]. The Infectious Disease Society of America, documented that management of several infectious diseases is extremely challenging such as vancomycin resistant *Enterococcus faccium*, multi-drug resistant *Acinetobacter baumannii*, methicillin-resistant *Staphylococcus aureus* (MRSA) and *Enterobacteriaecae* [19]. The development of antibiotic resistance occurs mainly due to gene mutation, horizontal gene transfers via conjugation, transformation and recombination events [20]. Broadly there are four mechanisms of multi-drug resistance in bacteria. They are:

- Modification of drug target;
- Drug inactivation;
- Drug target modification; and
- Bypass of target site.

Bacterial resistance leads to difficulty in treatment, causing serious complications in critically ill patients. These resistant bacteria spread not only in healthcare settings but also in communities [21]. Due to the limited options available for the treatment of infections caused by multi-drug resistant pathogens, there is an urgent need to explore new strategies to develop new drug candidates [22].

ROLE OF STRUCTURAL BIOLOGY IN DRUG DISCOVERY

Structure biology has a huge potential in drug discovery, structural information obtained from native structures of proteins and also their complexes with ligands can be used in designing of the lead compounds [23, 24]. Various industries utilize high-throughput and fragment screening approaches to identify the initial stage of small molecules in the research and development of drug discovery [25]. X-ray crystallography, electron crystallography, neutron crystallography, cryo-electron microscopy, small- angle neutron scattering and electron tomography are commonly used direct imaging techniques in structural biology for drug discovery [26 - 29]. Amongst these techniques, the ones which provide higher resolution in the structural determination of macromolecules complexes are X-ray crystallography, cryo-EM; hence are used more often in structural determination of target enzyme and their complexes with ligands (Table 1) [30].

On the basis of structural knowledge, three dimensional structure of macromolecules provides biological mechanisms and also suggests a new therapeutic mode for rational drug design [31, 32].

Table 1. Comparison of X-ray crystallography, NMR and Cryo-EM.

S. No.	X-ray Diffraction (XRD)	Nuclear Magnetic Resonance (NMR)	Cryo-EM
Technique	Involves arrangement of atoms within a crystal.	Involves change in nuclear spin energy in the presence of magnetic field.	Involves analysis of native structure in cryogenic condition which are sensitive towards radiation.
Based	Based on X-ray diffraction pattern.	Based on absorption or electromagnetic radiation in radio frequency range.	Based on native cryogenic condition.

(Table 1) cont.....

S. No.	X-ray Diffraction (XRD)	Nuclear Magnetic Resonance (NMR)	Cryo-EM
Resolution	High resolution	High resolution	Resolution is not high as compared to XRD and NMR.
Molecule size determination	No restriction of size	Relatively small protein molecule as compared to XRD	Large and complex protein structure can be determined.
Cost- effective	Relatively Cheap and simple technique.	Costly.	Costly.
Protein	Protein required in crystalline form.	Sample used in solution phase.	Frozen sample is used
Method	Static method	Dynamic method	Static method
Use	Useful for determining the 3-D structure of biological macromolecules.	Enhances our knowledge of protein such as folding and intra- intermolecular interactions, *etc.*	Useful for the structural study of large biological samples. (*e.g.,* virions, membrane proteins, *etc.*)
Limitation	Some biological macromolecules are difficult to crystallize (*e.g.* membrane proteins)	Cannot be used for determination of structure of large molecules.	Longer exposure of Electron beam can damage the sample. Large complexes give better results.

Drug targets are generally proteins and nucleic acids, which play an essential role in the survival of pathogen. Most often receptor proteins, metabolic enzymes, ion channels, membrane transport proteins and nucleic acids are recognized as drug targets. A good drug target should be essential for the survival of the pathogen, it should be unique as far as functional relevance is concerned, no other pathway should be able to supplement the function of the target and it should be druggable as its activity could be regulated by binding to a small molecule [24]. Various techniques are used for the identification of drug targets, including genetic polymorphism studies having a correlation with the disease, gene knockdown or knockout studies to directly explore the functional importance of the target, *in-vitro* studies for phenotypic analysis of the target, Expression profile studies to check the change in mRNA/protein expression level and structural bioinformatics approach for identifying of drug targets [11, 31]. Three dimensional models provide the information of families and super-families of protein which supports in identifying the binding sites or binding pockets and molecular functions. The profiling method is a powerful tool for recognition of homology performance by sequence structure comparison strategy [33]. After identification of homologue of known structure, it can be modelled by using bioinformatics tools. These homology model play a vital role in the development of inhibitors and successfully utilised as an initial point for *in silico* virtual screening. Hence, experimental approaches of bioinformatics with structural based function analogy is one of a method for drug targets identification (Fig. **1**) [34]. On the basis of a particular size, physiochemical properties and interaction with protein binding site, small molecules for drug target are designed [35]. Different databases are utilised for the identification of specific ligands interacting with the protein [36 - 39].

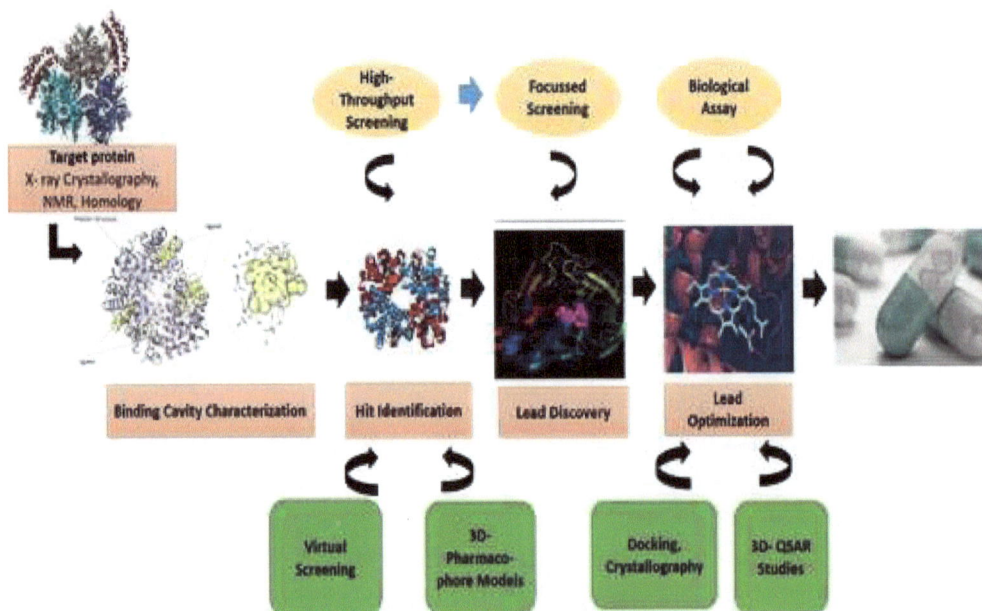

Fig. (1). Workflow of Structural Based Drug Design in Drug Discovery.

High throughput screening is one of the most effective approaches for lead identification. For the identification of lead molecules, new compound is selected with the help of previous knowledge of known identified ligands. Library of newly identified compounds are compared with the known ligand using different biophysical methods [40, 41]. X-ray crystallography screening has great advantage in identifying ligand and confirming the binding of the ligand to the protein based on the presence of electron density of the ligand at the active site [53]. Biophysical affinity based methods are able to provide kinetic and thermodynamics parameters, which recognize equilibrium binding and measurement of affinity, to improve the success during hit to lead transformation [42]. Combined studies of kinetic and thermodynamics with high quality structural data provide the best information to enhance our understanding of protein-ligand interactions natures [43].

While optimization of lead compounds, Potency, Selectivity and ADME properties are considered. Structural based drug design and fragment based drug design are performed, which provide information about the lead compound [44].

X-RAY CRYSTALLOGRAPHY AND COMPUTATIONAL METHODS FOR LIGAND SCREENING IN DRUG DISCOVERY

X-ray crystallography is a comprehensive technique that provide overall information about the conformation and structure of any molecule at atomic resolutions [46 - 48]. It is the most accurate, precise and reliable technique which generates accurate image of protein in hydration state in the crystal form [49]. Structures are evaluated on the basis of experimental diffraction pattern, analysis of electron density and their functional mechanism [50]. For determining the three-dimension structure of the protein, X-ray crystallography provides high resolution macromolecule structure that can also be utilised to establish large heteromeric complexes such as ribosomes and provide the complete information of experimental affirmation of the binding mode of ligands, which is found in the crystals [37, 51 - 53].

X-ray crystallography has emerged as a powerful ligand screening technique for determining the structural information of protein ligand complexes [42]. On the basis of the structural information derived from the protein, ligands are designed which can bind protein with increased affinity [51]. Ligands can be designed on the basis of previously known molecules that binds to the protein or architecture of the binding pocket of the protein. Moreover, by this process whole fragment library can be screened which provide the detailed structural information of ligand and target interaction in drug process [42, 50]. The ligands showing the best affinity with the protein can be validated by different biophysical activity and inhibition assays in the case of enzymes.

De novo ligand based drug design and Virtual screening are the computational methods for ligand screening in drug discovery (Fig. **2**) [54 - 56]. *De novo* ligand based drug design are low cost and time-efficient molecular optimization methods, which can help in developing novel drug candidates with desired properties [57, 58]. Fragment positioning methods, molecular growing and fragment methods are the three classes of *De novo* ligand based drug design. Cyclophilin A inhibitor is a successful example of *de novo* drug design using LigBuilder 2.0 [59]. Virtual screening has proved itself a successful cost effective technique that works on the basis of high binding affinity of the ligand to protein target by using virtual compound libraries. Virtual screening consists of Molecular docking, Quantitative Structure-Activity Relationship (QSAR) and Pharmacophore modelling, *etc.* [60, 61].

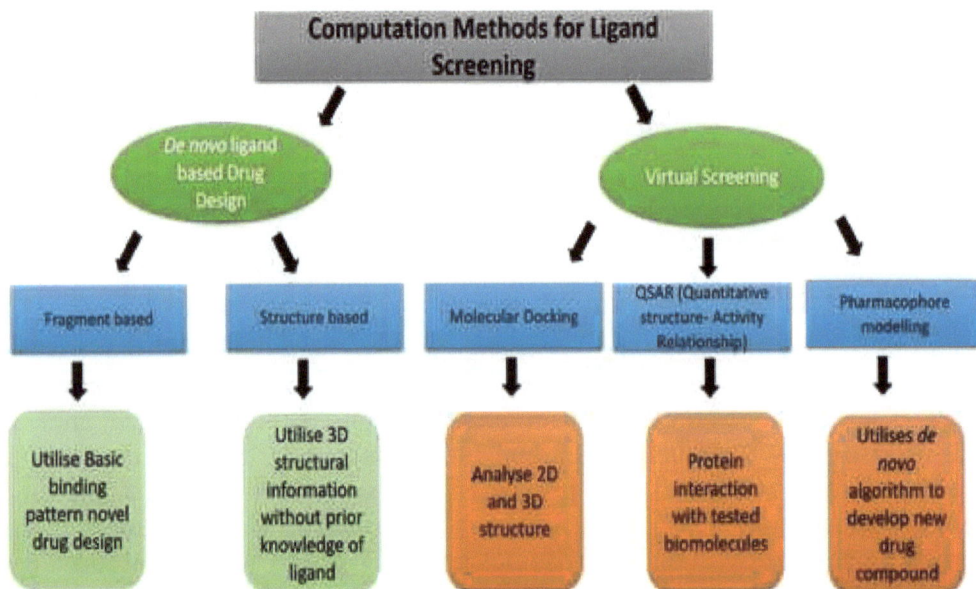

Fig. (2). Computation methods for ligand screening.

CHALLENGES AND STRATEGIES FOR TREATMENT OF MULTI DRUG RESISTANT INFECTIONS

Multi-drug resistant strains are characterized as "Crisis" in several health organizations [62]. Failure of antibiotics in the treatment of multi-drug resistant infections is currently one of the most alarming concern in healthcare settings. The main reason behind the failure of antibiotic is because microbes are not able to respond to standard drugs (Fig. **3**) [63]. Tolerance, persistence and resistance are the three different mechanisms of antimicrobial activity of antibiotics, which can be evaded by bacteria [64]. The ESKAPE are the most common opportunistic pathogens consisting of *Enterococcus faecium, Staphylococcus aureus*, Klebsiella pneumonia, Acinetobacter baumannii, *Pseudomonas aeruginosa* and *Enterobacter* species. The group of six multi-drug resistant pathogens (ESKAPE) are responsible for life threatening nosocomial infections and prolonged duration of treatment course [65]. ESKAPE pathogens are different from normal microbes because of their high level of multi-drug resistance, which includes multiple mechanisms [66]. Due to several mechanisms of antimicrobial resistance and narrow- spectrum drug targets of ESKAPE pathogens developed as major therapeutic challenges [67]. Long duration of illness, high medical cost, transmissibility, low efficiency of drugs, limited therapeutic options, prevention barriers and easy target for immunocompromised patients are the problems associated with multidrug resistant infections [68].

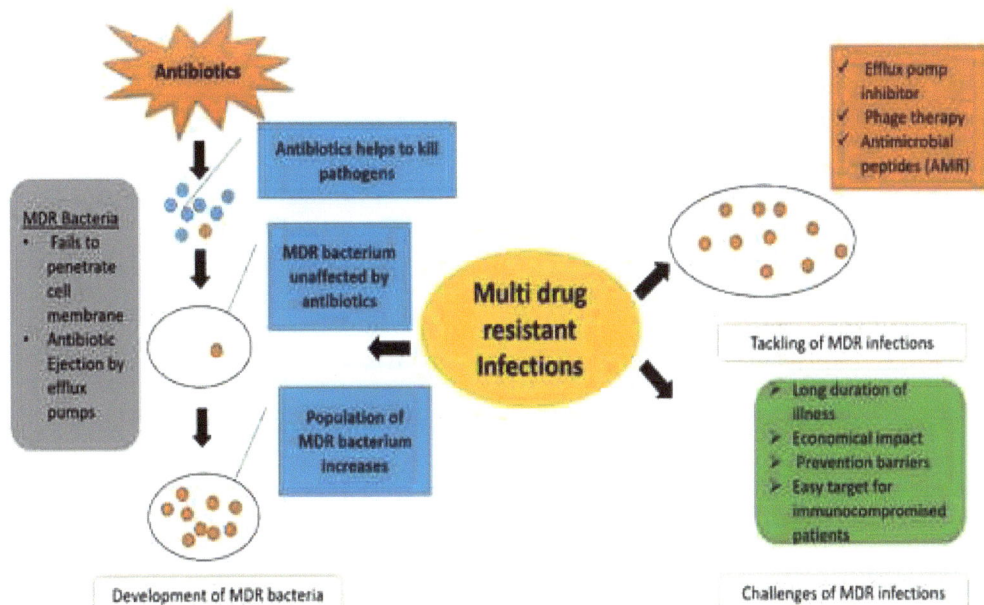

Fig. (3). Multi- drug resistant infections.

To control the development of bacterial resistance against antimicrobial, there are several strategies for the identification of novel drug targets which are focused on inhibiting the virulence-associated proteins [69]. Targeting bacterial pathways which are responsible for the survival of bacteria employs significant pressure that enhance the emergence of antibiotic resistant strains [70]. New therapies and drug repurposing are also anti-infectious strategies for tackling multidrug resistant bacteria. New therapies consist of antimicrobial peptides (AMPs) including biofilm inhibitors, phage therapies, anti-virluence and drug repurposing includes FDA approved drugs such as anti-inflammatory, anti-helmintics, anti-psychotic and anti-cancerous [71].

Antimicrobial Peptides (AMPs)

AMPs are positively charged host defence oligopeptides, developed for the treatment of multi-drug resistant infections. They have a broad range of antimicrobial activity and the ability to reduce the emergence of resistance [72]. It is a promising strategy to tackle multi-drug resistant bacteria by damaging the bacterial cell wall physically through electrostatic interaction. AMPs are a promising approach against ESKAPE pathogens [73]. Polymaxin, bacitracin, daptomycin and gramicidin are some examples of AMPs as a drug candidates [74].

Phage Therapies

Phage therapy is an alternative antibacterial strategy to combat the spread of multi-drug resistant organisms. They include lytic virus as a drug that interact with host immune system and kills the pathogenic bacteria to treat several infectious diseases [71, 75]. Phage therapy is an ideal approach to prevent multi-drug resistant infections because of high host specificity and rapid escalation inside the host cells. The combination of phage with drug can be a suitable option to tackle multi-drug resistant organism [76].

Quorum Sensing (QS) and Efflux Pump Inhibitors

QS inhibitors and efflux pump inhibitors can control the infections caused by multi-drug resistant bacteria [77]. Combination of Acyldepsipeptide antibiotic and rifampicin can completely disrupt the formation of biofilm. AcrAB- ToIC is an example of efflux pump inhibitor that could reactivate the sensitivity of antibiotic as well as restore the rate of mutation in *E. coli*. These compounds inhibit the growth of bacteria and can enhance the current treatment against multi-drug resistant infections [78, 79]. Anti- inflammatory, anti-helmintics, anti- psychotic and anti-cancerous are the anti-bacterial agents that are well defined in strategies of repurposing FDA approved drugs for the treatment against infections [71].

Structural based drug design has become a prevailing strategy to develop novel drug using information obtained from three-dimensional structure of proteins [80]. Drugs molecule obtained by structural based drug design inhibit the virulence-associated proteins, which are responsible for the survival of the pathogen and play a crucial role in their metabolic pathways. They do not affect humans and assist in the treatment of multi-drug resistant infections [38]. By using angiotensin- converting enzyme inhibitor, Captopril is the first derived drug from structure based drug design approach, which commonly used for hypertension and heart failure [81]. Dorzolamide and saquinavir are some successful examples of structural based drug design [46, 82].

CONCLUSION

The methods and strategies discussed in this chapter highlight the drug discovery for multi-drug resistant pathogens. Although, there are challenges for treatment of multi-drug resistant infections due to the limited therapeutic options. But rational structure based drug design approach can be successfully applied for the identification of new drug targets against multi-drug resistant infections. It is an efficient, cost effective and time saving approach to develop new drug targets. Rational structure based drug design is a multidisciplinary approach to develop drugs on the basis of 3-dimensional structures of the target molecules. Tertiary structures of proteins are determined by X-ray crystallography and NMR, which contributed to drug discovery and development in late stage clinical trial compounds. X-ray crystallography emerged as the most accurate and precise technique, which provides a high resolution for determining the tertiary structure of protein. Structure biology has a huge potential for drug discovery. It plays a crucial role in the identification of drug targets, assessment of drug targets, lead identification and lead discovery. Computational methods can accelerate the development of drugs and recognize highly efficient therapies and mechanism of action that can be applied to a variety of biological systems.

CONSENT FOR PUBLICATION

Not applicable.

CONFLICT OF INTEREST

The authors declare no conflict of interest, financial or otherwise.

ACKNOWLEDGEMENTS

Declared none.

REFERENCES

[1]   Zaman SB, Hussain MA, Nye R, Mehta V, Mamun KT, Hossain N. A review on antibiotic resistance: alarm bells are ringing. Cureus 2017; 9(6): e1403.
[http://dx.doi.org/10.7759/cureus.1403] [PMID: 28852600]

[2]   Raghunath D. Emerging antibiotic resistance in bacteria with special reference to India. J Biosci 2008; 33(4): 593-603.
[http://dx.doi.org/10.1007/s12038-008-0077-9] [PMID: 19208984]

[3]   Medina E, Pieper DH. Tackling threats and future problems of multidrug-resistant bacteria. Curr Top Microbiol Immunol 2016; 398: 3-33.
[http://dx.doi.org/10.1007/82_2016_492]

[4]   Holmes AH, Moore LS, Sundsfjord A, *et al.* Understanding the mechanisms and drivers of antimicrobial resistance. Lancet 2016; 387(10014): 176-87.
[http://dx.doi.org/10.1016/S0140-6736(15)00473-0] [PMID: 26603922]

[5]   Martins M, McCusker MP, Viveiros M, *et al.* A simple method for assessment of MDR bacteria for over-expressed efflux pumps. Open Microbiol J 2013; 7: 72-82.
[http://dx.doi.org/10.2174/1874285801307010072] [PMID: 23589748]

[6]   Vernon JJ. Multidrug Resistant Clostridioides difficile: The Presence of Antimicrobial Resistance Determinants in Historical and Contemporaneous Isolates, and the Impact of Fluoroquinolone Resistance Development. Doctoral dissertation, The University of Leeds

[7]   Simões M, Bennett RN, Rosa EA. Understanding antimicrobial activities of phytochemicals against multidrug resistant bacteria and biofilms. Nat Prod Rep 2009; 26(6): 746-57.
[http://dx.doi.org/10.1039/b821648g] [PMID: 19471683]

[8]   Abolghait SK, Fathi AG, Youssef FM, Algammal AM. Methicillin-resistant *Staphylococcus aureus* (MRSA) isolated from chicken meat and giblets often produces staphylococcal enterotoxin B (SEB) in

non-refrigerated raw chicken livers. Int J Food Microbiol 2020; 328: 108669.
[http://dx.doi.org/10.1016/j.ijfoodmicro.2020.108669] [PMID: 32497922]

[9] Cetinkaya Y, Falk P, Mayhall CG. Vancomycin-resistant enterococci. Clin Microbiol Rev 2000; 13(4): 686-707.
[http://dx.doi.org/10.1128/CMR.13.4.686] [PMID: 11023964]

[10] Magiorakos AP, Srinivasan A, Carey RB, *et al.* Multidrug-resistant, extensively drug-resistant and pandrug-resistant bacteria: an international expert proposal for interim standard definitions for acquired resistance. Clin Microbiol Infect 2012; 18(3): 268-81.
[http://dx.doi.org/10.1111/j.1469-0691.2011.03570.x] [PMID: 21793988]

[11] Prabhakar B, Zhong XB, Rasmussen TP. Focus: drug development: exploiting long noncoding RNAs as pharmacological targets to modulate epigenetic diseases. Yale J Biol Med 2017; 90(1): 73-86.
[PMID: 28356895]

[12] Penchovsky R, Traykovska M. Designing drugs that overcome antibacterial resistance: where do we stand and what should we do? Expert Opin Drug Discov 2015; 10(6): 631-50.
[http://dx.doi.org/10.1517/17460441.2015.1048219] [PMID: 25981754]

[13] Ferreira LG, Dos Santos RN, Oliva G, Andricopulo AD. Molecular docking and structure-based drug design strategies. Molecules 2015; 20(7): 13384-421.
[http://dx.doi.org/10.3390/molecules200713384] [PMID: 26205061]

[14] Vénien-Bryan C, Li Z, Vuillard L, Boutin JA. Cryo-electron microscopy and X-ray crystallography: complementary approaches to structural biology and drug discovery. Acta Crystallogr F Struct Biol Commun 2017; 73(Pt 4): 174-83.
[http://dx.doi.org/10.1107/S2053230X17003740] [PMID: 28368275]

[15] Milne JL, Borgnia MJ, Bartesaghi A, *et al.* Cryo-electron microscopy--a primer for the non-microscopist. FEBS J 2013; 280(1): 28-45.
[http://dx.doi.org/10.1111/febs.12078] [PMID: 23181775]

[16] Wang X, Song K, Li L, Chen L. Structure-based drug design strategies and challenges. Curr Top Med Chem 2018; 18(12): 998-1006.
[http://dx.doi.org/10.2174/1568026618666180813152921] [PMID: 30101712]

[17] Lye DC, Earnest A, Ling ML, *et al.* The impact of multidrug resistance in healthcare-associated and nosocomial Gram-negative bacteraemia on mortality and length of stay: cohort study. Clin Microbiol Infect 2012; 18(5): 502-8.
[http://dx.doi.org/10.1111/j.1469-0691.2011.03606.x] [PMID: 21851482]

[18] Pal C, Bengtsson-Palme J, Kristiansson E, Larsson DG. Co-occurrence of resistance genes to antibiotics, biocides and metals reveals novel insights into their co-selection potential. BMC Genomics 2015; 16: 964.
[http://dx.doi.org/10.1186/s12864-015-2153-5] [PMID: 26576951]

[19] Talbot GH, Bradley J, Edwards JE Jr, Gilbert D, Scheld M, Bartlett JG. Bad bugs need drugs: an update on the development pipeline from the Antimicrobial Availability Task Force of the Infectious Diseases Society of America. Clin Infect Dis 2006; 42(5): 657-68.
[http://dx.doi.org/10.1086/499819] [PMID: 16447111]

[20] Schmidt T, Bergner A, Schwede T. Modelling three-dimensional protein structures for applications in drug design. Drug Discov Today 2014; 19(7): 890-7.
[http://dx.doi.org/10.1016/j.drudis.2013.10.027] [PMID: 24216321]

[21] Livermore DM. Bacterial resistance: origins, epidemiology, and impact. Clin Infect Dis 2003; 36 (Suppl. 1): S11-23.
[http://dx.doi.org/10.1086/344654] [PMID: 12516026]

[22] Brown ED, Wright GD. Antibacterial drug discovery in the resistance era. Nature 2016; 529(7586): 336-43.

[http://dx.doi.org/10.1038/nature17042] [PMID: 26791724]

[23]   Mortier J, Rakers C, Bermudez M, Murgueitio MS, Riniker S, Wolber G. The impact of molecular dynamics on drug design: applications for the characterization of ligand-macromolecule complexes. Drug Discov Today 2015; 20(6): 686-702.
[http://dx.doi.org/10.1016/j.drudis.2015.01.003] [PMID: 25615716]

[24]   Renaud JP, Chung CW, Danielson UH, *et al.* Biophysics in drug discovery: impact, challenges and opportunities. Nat Rev Drug Discov 2016; 15(10): 679-98.
[http://dx.doi.org/10.1038/nrd.2016.123] [PMID: 27516170]

[25]   Macarron R, Banks MN, Bojanic D, *et al.* Impact of high-throughput screening in biomedical research. Nat Rev Drug Discov 2011; 10(3): 188-95.
[http://dx.doi.org/10.1038/nrd3368] [PMID: 21358738]

[26]   Petoukhov MV, Svergun DI. Analysis of X-ray and neutron scattering from biomacromolecular solutions. Curr Opin Struct Biol 2007; 17(5): 562-71.
[http://dx.doi.org/10.1016/j.sbi.2007.06.009] [PMID: 17714935]

[27]   Nogales E, Scheres SH. Cryo-EM: a unique tool for the visualization of macromolecular complexity. Mol Cell 2015; 58(4): 677-89.
[http://dx.doi.org/10.1016/j.molcel.2015.02.019] [PMID: 26000851]

[28]   Fan Y, Wang Y. Applications of small-angle X-ray scattering/small-angle neutron scattering and cryogenic transmission electron microscopy to understand self-assembly of surfactants. Curr Opin Colloid In 2019; 42: 1-6.
[http://dx.doi.org/10.1016/j.cocis.2019.02.011]

[29]   Renaud JP. Structural Biology in Drug Discovery. Wiley 2020.
[http://dx.doi.org/10.1002/9781118681121]

[30]   Bai XC, McMullan G, Scheres SH. How cryo-EM is revolutionizing structural biology. Trends Biochem Sci 2015; 40(1): 49-57.
[http://dx.doi.org/10.1016/j.tibs.2014.10.005] [PMID: 25544475]

[31]   Yang GF, Huang X. Development of quantitative structure-activity relationships and its application in rational drug design. Curr Pharm Des 2006; 12(35): 4601-11.
[http://dx.doi.org/10.2174/138161206779010431] [PMID: 17168765]

[32]   Kalyaanamoorthy S, Chen YP. Structure-based drug design to augment hit discovery. Drug Discov Today 2011; 16(17-18): 831-9.
[http://dx.doi.org/10.1016/j.drudis.2011.07.006] [PMID: 21810482]

[33]   Blundell TL, Sibanda BL, Montalvão RW, *et al.* Structural biology and bioinformatics in drug design: opportunities and challenges for target identification and lead discovery. Philos Trans R Soc Lond B Biol Sci 2006; 361(1467): 413-23.
[http://dx.doi.org/10.1098/rstb.2005.1800] [PMID: 16524830]

[34]   Scapin G. Structural biology and drug discovery. Curr Pharm Des 2006; 12(17): 2087-97.
[http://dx.doi.org/10.2174/138161206777585201] [PMID: 16796557]

[35]   Scott DE, Bayly AR, Abell C, Skidmore J. Small molecules, big targets: drug discovery faces the protein-protein interaction challenge. Nat Rev Drug Discov 2016; 15(8): 533-50.
[http://dx.doi.org/10.1038/nrd.2016.29] [PMID: 27050677]

[36]   Volkamer A, Kuhn D, Grombacher T, Rippmann F, Rarey M. Combining global and local measures for structure-based druggability predictions. J Chem Inf Model 2012; 52(2): 360-72.
[http://dx.doi.org/10.1021/ci200454v] [PMID: 22148551]

[37]   Zheng H, Hou J, Zimmerman MD, Wlodawer A, Minor W. The future of crystallography in drug discovery. Expert Opin Drug Discov 2014; 9(2): 125-37.
[http://dx.doi.org/10.1517/17460441.2014.872623] [PMID: 24372145]

[38] Jubb H, Higueruelo AP, Winter A, Blundell TL. Structural biology and drug discovery for protein-protein interactions. Trends Pharmacol Sci 2012; 33(5): 241-8.
[http://dx.doi.org/10.1016/j.tips.2012.03.006] [PMID: 22503442]

[39] Tradigo G, Rondinelli F, Pollastri G. Algorithms for structure comparison and analysis: Docking. Encyclopedia of Bioinformatics and Computational Biology: ABC of Bioinformatics. 2018; 77.

[40] Batool M, Ahmad B, Choi S. A structure-based drug discovery paradigm. Int J Mol Sci 2019; 20(11): 2783.
[http://dx.doi.org/10.3390/ijms20112783] [PMID: 31174387]

[41] Rondeau JM, Schreuder H. Protein crystallography and drug discovery. The practice of medicinal chemistry. Academic Press 2008; pp. 605-34.
[http://dx.doi.org/10.1016/B978-0-12-374194-3.00030-5]

[42] Maveyraud L, Mourey L. Protein X-ray Crystallography and Drug Discovery. Molecules 2020; 25(5): 1030.
[http://dx.doi.org/10.3390/molecules25051030] [PMID: 32106588]

[43] Spiliopoulou M, Valmas A, Triandafillidis DP, *et al.* Applications of X-ray powder diffraction in protein crystallography and drug screening. Crystals (Basel) 2020; 10: 54.
[http://dx.doi.org/10.3390/cryst10020054]

[44] Leach AR, Hann MM. Introduction to Fragment Screening InStructure-Based Drug Discovery. Dordrecht: Springer 2007; pp. 49-72.

[45] Patwardhan A, Brandt R, Butcher SJ, *et al.* Building bridges between cellular and molecular structural biology. eLife 2017; 6: e25835.
[http://dx.doi.org/10.7554/eLife.25835] [PMID: 28682240]

[46] Blundell TL, Patel S. High-throughput X-ray crystallography for drug discovery. Curr Opin Pharmacol 2004; 4(5): 490-6.
[http://dx.doi.org/10.1016/j.coph.2004.04.007] [PMID: 15351354]

[47] Flack HD, Bernardinelli G. The use of X-ray crystallography to determine absolute configuration. Pharmacological, Biological, and Chemical Consequences of Molecular Asymmetry 2008; 20(5): 681-90.
[http://dx.doi.org/10.1002/chir.20473] [PMID: 17924422]

[48] Deschamps JR. The role of crystallography in drug design. Drug Addiction 2008; pp. 343-55.
[http://dx.doi.org/10.1007/978-0-387-76678-2_21]

[49] Lounnas V, Ritschel T, Kelder J, McGuire R, Bywater RP, Foloppe N. Current progress in Structure-Based Rational Drug Design marks a new mindset in drug discovery. Comput Struct Biotechnol J 2013; 5: e201302011.
[http://dx.doi.org/10.5936/csbj.201302011] [PMID: 24688704]

[50] Carvalho AL, Trincão J, Romão MJ. X-ray crystallography in drug discovery. Ligand-Macromolecular Interactions in Drug Discovery 2010; pp. 31-56.

[51] Livingston DA, Buchanan SG, D'Amico KL, Milburn MV, Peat TS, Sauder JM. X-Ray Crystallography in Drug Discovery. Burger's Med Chem Drug Discov 2003; pp. 611-32.

[52] Acharya KR, Lloyd MD. The advantages and limitations of protein crystal structures. Trends Pharmacol Sci 2005; 26(1): 10-4.
[http://dx.doi.org/10.1016/j.tips.2004.10.011] [PMID: 15629199]

[53] Thompson AL, Watkin DJ. X-ray crystallography and chirality: understanding the limitations. Tetrahedron Asymmetry 2009; 20: 712-7.
[http://dx.doi.org/10.1016/j.tetasy.2009.02.025]

[54] Fader KA, Zhang J, Menetski JP, *et al.* A Biomarker-Centric Approach to Drug Discovery and Development: Lessons Learned from the Coronavirus Disease 2019 Pandemic. J Pharmacol Exp Ther

2021; 376(1): 12-20.
[http://dx.doi.org/10.1124/jpet.120.000204] [PMID: 33115823]

[55]   Anwar T, Kumar P, Khan AU. Modern Tools and Techniques in Computer-Aided Drug Design. Molecular Docking for Computer-Aided Drug Design. Academic Press 2021; pp. 1-30.
[http://dx.doi.org/10.1016/B978-0-12-822312-3.00011-4]

[56]   Wang Z, Sun H, Shen C, *et al.* Combined strategies in structure-based virtual screening. Phys Chem Chem Phys 2020; 22(6): 3149-59.
[http://dx.doi.org/10.1039/C9CP06303J] [PMID: 31995074]

[57]   Devi RV, Sathya SS, Coumar MS. Evolutionary algorithms for de novo drug design–A survey. Appl Soft Comput 2015; 27: 543-52.
[http://dx.doi.org/10.1016/j.asoc.2014.09.042]

[58]   Krishnan SR, Bung N, Bulusu G, Roy A. Accelerating de novo drug design against novel proteins using deep learning. J Chem Inf Model 2021; 61(2): 621-30.
[http://dx.doi.org/10.1021/acs.jcim.0c01060] [PMID: 33491455]

[59]   Ni S, Yuan Y, Huang J, *et al.* Discovering potent small molecule inhibitors of cyclophilin A using *de novo* drug design approach. J Med Chem 2009; 52(17): 5295-8.
[http://dx.doi.org/10.1021/jm9008295] [PMID: 19691347]

[60]   Sliwoski G, Kothiwale S, Meiler J, Lowe EW Jr. Computational methods in drug discovery. Pharmacol Rev 2013; 66(1): 334-95.
[http://dx.doi.org/10.1124/pr.112.007336] [PMID: 24381236]

[61]   Lin X, Li X, Lin X. A review on applications of computational methods in drug screening and design. Molecules 2020; 25(6): 1375.
[http://dx.doi.org/10.3390/molecules25061375] [PMID: 32197324]

[62]   Perez F, Hujer AM, Hujer KM, Decker BK, Rather PN, Bonomo RA. Global challenge of multidrug-resistant Acinetobacter baumannii. Antimicrob Agents Chemother 2007; 51(10): 3471-84.
[http://dx.doi.org/10.1128/AAC.01464-06] [PMID: 17646423]

[63]   Mulvey MR, Simor AE. Antimicrobial resistance in hospitals: how concerned should we be? CMAJ 2009; 180(4): 408-15.
[http://dx.doi.org/10.1503/cmaj.080239] [PMID: 19221354]

[64]   Balaban NQ, Helaine S, Lewis K, *et al.* Definitions and guidelines for research on antibiotic persistence. Nat Rev Microbiol 2019; 17(7): 441-8.
[http://dx.doi.org/10.1038/s41579-019-0196-3] [PMID: 30980069]

[65]   Pendleton JN, Gorman SP, Gilmore BF. Clinical relevance of the ESKAPE pathogens. Expert Rev Anti Infect Ther 2013; 11(3): 297-308.
[http://dx.doi.org/10.1586/eri.13.12] [PMID: 23458769]

[66]   Santajit S, Indrawattana N. Mechanisms of antimicrobial resistance in ESKAPE pathogens. BioMed Res Int 2016.
[http://dx.doi.org/10.1155/2016/2475067]

[67]   Mulani MS, Kamble EE, Kumkar SN, Tawre MS, Pardesi KR. Emerging strategies to combat ESKAPE pathogens in the era of antimicrobial resistance: a review. Front Microbiol 2019; 10: 539.
[http://dx.doi.org/10.3389/fmicb.2019.00539] [PMID: 30988669]

[68]   Mukherjee JS, Rich ML, Socci AR, *et al.* Programmes and principles in treatment of multidrug-resistant tuberculosis. Lancet 2004; 363(9407): 474-81.
[http://dx.doi.org/10.1016/S0140-6736(04)15496-2] [PMID: 14962530]

[69]   Gill EE, Franco OL, Hancock RE. Antibiotic adjuvants: diverse strategies for controlling drug-resistant pathogens. Chem Biol Drug Des 2015; 85(1): 56-78.
[http://dx.doi.org/10.1111/cbdd.12478] [PMID: 25393203]

[70] Petchiappan A, Chatterji D. Antibiotic resistance: current perspectives. ACS Omega 2017; 2(10): 7400-9.
[http://dx.doi.org/10.1021/acsomega.7b01368] [PMID: 30023551]

[71] Pacios O, Blasco L, Bleriot I, *et al*. Strategies to combat multidrug-resistant and persistent infectious diseases. Antibiotics (Basel) 2020; 9(2): 65.
[http://dx.doi.org/10.3390/antibiotics9020065] [PMID: 32041137]

[72] Park SC, Park Y, Hahm KS. The role of antimicrobial peptides in preventing multidrug-resistant bacterial infections and biofilm formation. Int J Mol Sci 2011; 12(9): 5971-92.
[http://dx.doi.org/10.3390/ijms12095971] [PMID: 22016639]

[73] Lam SJ, O'Brien-Simpson NM, Pantarat N, *et al*. Combating multidrug-resistant Gram-negative bacteria with structurally nanoengineered antimicrobial peptide polymers. Nat Microbiol 2016; 1(11): 16162.
[http://dx.doi.org/10.1038/nmicrobiol.2016.162] [PMID: 27617798]

[74] Costa F, Teixeira C, Gomes P, Martins MC. Clinical application of AMPs. Antimicrobial Peptides 2019; pp. 281-98.

[75] Golkar Z, Bagasra O, Pace DG. Bacteriophage therapy: a potential solution for the antibiotic resistance crisis. J Infect Dev Ctries 2014; 8(2): 129-36.
[http://dx.doi.org/10.3855/jidc.3573] [PMID: 24518621]

[76] Kortright KE, Chan BK, Koff JL, Turner PE. Phage therapy: a renewed approach to combat antibiotic-resistant bacteria. Cell Host Microbe 2019; 25(2): 219-32.
[http://dx.doi.org/10.1016/j.chom.2019.01.014] [PMID: 30763536]

[77] Subhadra B, Kim DH, Woo K, Surendran S, Choi CH. Control of biofilm formation in healthcare: Recent advances exploiting quorum-sensing interference strategies and multidrug efflux pump inhibitors. Materials (Basel) 2018; 11(9): 1676.
[http://dx.doi.org/10.3390/ma11091676] [PMID: 30201944]

[78] Álvarez-Martínez FJ, Barrajón-Catalán E, Micol V. Tackling antibiotic resistance with compounds of natural origin: A comprehensive review. Biomedicines 2020; 8(10): 405.
[http://dx.doi.org/10.3390/biomedicines8100405] [PMID: 33050619]

[79] Ricci V, Blair JM, Piddock LJ. RamA, which controls expression of the MDR efflux pump AcrAB-TolC, is regulated by the Lon protease. J Antimicrob Chemother 2014; 69(3): 643-50.
[http://dx.doi.org/10.1093/jac/dkt432] [PMID: 24169580]

[80] Veerapandian P, Ed. Structure-based drug design. Routledge 2018.
[http://dx.doi.org/10.1201/9780203738023]

[81] Cushman DW, Ondetti MA. History of the design of captopril and related inhibitors of angiotensin converting enzyme. Hypertension 1991; 17(4): 589-92.
[http://dx.doi.org/10.1161/01.HYP.17.4.589] [PMID: 2013486]

[82] Kroemer RT. Structure-based drug design: docking and scoring. Curr Protein Pept Sci 2007; 8(4): 312-28.
[http://dx.doi.org/10.2174/138920307781369382] [PMID: 17696866]

CHAPTER 11

Recent Developments to Fight Multidrug Resistance (MDR) in Protozoa

Mrinalini Roy[1], Sanket Kaushik[1], Anupam Jyoti[2] and **Vijay Kumar Srivastava[1,*]**

[1] *Amity Institute of Biotechnology, Amity University Rajasthan, Kant Kalwar, NH-11C, Jaipur-Delhi Highway, Jaipur, India*

[2] *Department of Biotechnology, University Institute of Biotechnology, Chandigarh University, NH-95, Chandigarh-Ludhiana Highway, Mohali, India*

Abstract: This chapter focuses on the solutions to emerging multidrug resistance in the major parasitic protozoa plaguing the world. These neglected pathogens have seized the developing nations in a vice-like grip and are seeping into the industrialised world with the dramatic increase in global travel. The alarming rise in resistance to most antiparasitic drugs has left even the wealthiest nations vulnerable. Multidrug resistance occurs to give a survival advantage to the parasite; it has been hastened by the uncontrolled use of chemotherapeutics. This chapter categorises the recent developments to overcome the MDR hurdle under different approaches. The synthesis of novel organic compounds and high-throughput screenings of new chemical entities are two major approaches. Protease and topoisomerase inhibitors of parasitic protozoa prove as worthy drug targets. *In-silico* and proteomics-based methods also accelerate drug discovery by creating potential drug libraries specific to tropical protozoa. A cost-effective and rapid method of combating drug resistance is the repurposing of licensed medicines. This approach also accounts for the established safety of drugs and high commercial availability. Molecular advancements have introduced small interfering RNAs (siRNAs) at preclinical levels as therapeutics functioning *via* a unique mechanism. The nanoparticle and cell-penetrating peptides (CPP) based delivery of siRNAs has facilitated a stable and low toxic way to silence genes providing pathogenicity and resistance. This will help in reversing MDR and breathing new life into the existing licensed antiprotozoal chemotherapies.

Keywords: Antimicrobial peptides, Antiprotozoal therapeutics, Aystems biology, Drug repurposing, *In-silico*, Multidrug resistance, Protease inhibitors, siRNA, Synthetic organic compounds.

* Corresponding author Vijay Kumar Srivastava: Amity Institute of Biotechnology, Amity University Rajasthan, Kant Kalwar, NH-11C, Jaipur-Delhi Highway, Jaipur, India; E-mail: vksrivastava@jpr.amity.edu

Sanket Kaushik and Nagendra Singh (Eds.)
All rights reserved-© 2022 Bentham Science Publishers

INTRODUCTION

The blight of protozoan disease is no longer limited to developing and poor nations; it has found a hold in the industrialised world as well due to increased global travel and multidrug resistance. Multidrug resistance (MDR) is defined as the insensitivity of an organism to the administered chemotherapeutics (that have different molecular targets) despite earlier sensitivity to it.

The fitness model of natural evolution promotes MDR. The phenomenon has accelerated in the last two decades with extensive and unnecessary use of chemotherapy. This situation is further complicated by incomplete clearance of pathogens because of viral and lifestyle-induced immune-insufficiency, which creates recalcitrant and recurring infections. The vicious cycle of resistance fuels the further spread of MDR as a consequence of chronic infections and long term hospitalisations that enable hospital-acquired infections to become a hotspot for the exchange of resistance mechanisms between parasites [1].

Pathogenic protozoa have created several MDR adaptations. These include rapid efflux of the drug and the reduction in drug uptake due to modifications in drug transporters. These transporters often hide in plain sight under other simplistic functions. Drug modification, drug degradation and sequestration, genetic mutations and target enzyme modulations, all augment MDR. These mechanisms are illustrated in Fig. (**1**). Thus, it is essential to formulate nontoxic and cost-effective chemotherapies for managing protozoan infections. Moreover, the new drugs should be mechanistically novel so that existing resistance mechanisms do not render the new drugs ineffective [2, 3].

Scientific and political advancements in developing nations have helped alleviate the obstacles in the drug discovery against parasitic protozoa. A multidisciplinary approach based on structural studies of protozoal proteins, genomic analysis and high-throughput screening of compound libraries has driven this change. In this chapter, you will learn about the recent developments in antiprotozoal therapies to overcome the multidrug resistance to conventional treatments in major pathogenic protozoa.

NEWLY SYNTHESIZED ORGANIC COMPOUNDS

Researchers have accumulated data about parasitic biochemistry over the last half-century to develop antiprotozoal drugs. They have used this biochemical data to synthesize organic molecules that block the parasitic activities of protozoa [4]. Some of these are first-line drugs, such as metronidazole for gastric protozoa, and pentavalent antimonials for leishmaniasis. However, most conventional drugs are increasingly becoming redundant with the emergence of multidrug resistance [5].

The decades of data from protozoan pathogenicity and metabolomic studies have brought to light, new targets for drug discovery. The researchers have exploited this knowledge to synthesize new organic compounds to launch mechanistically novel drugs in the market. All the new formulations have been compared to standard drugs to check for efficacy and toxicity, before declaring them as potential antiprotozoal therapies [6, 7].

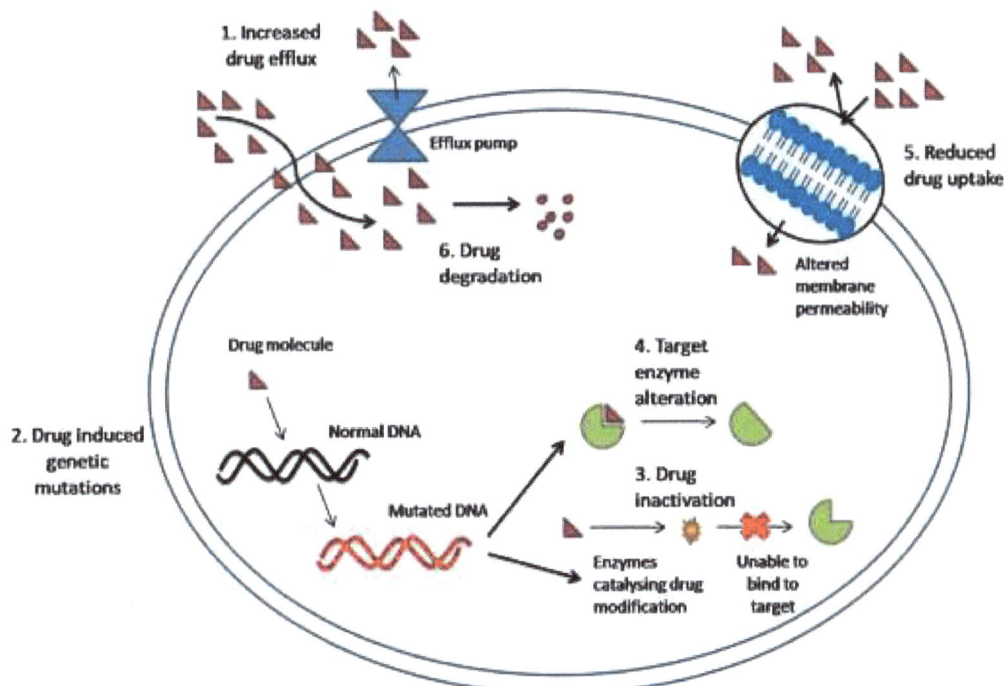

Fig. (1). Schematic diagram of mechanisms of MDR.

Different series of heterocyclic compounds have been studied and their derivatives were synthesized. Among these, a hybrid compound designed by linking molecular scaffolds of pyrazoline and pyrimidine showed excellent activity against *Leishmania donovani* and *Leishmania major* [8]. The Drugs for Neglected Diseases *initiative* (DND*i*) has introduced a highly effective aminopyrazole series for the treatment of visceral and cutaneous leishmaniasis. The aminopyrazole based medicines were not affected by the activity of MDR efflux pumps thus exhibiting a low potential for resistance [9]. The series of 1,3-dipyridylbenzene and terphenyl diamide derivatives revealed good drug candidates against *Trypanosoma brucei rhodesiense* and *Trypanosoma cruzi* strains with IC_{50} values comparable to the standard drug, melarsoprol. Low IC_{50} values of 0.16 µM and 0.10 µM were displayed by two imidazolic compounds, against human African trypanosomiasis (HAT) or sleeping sickness [10, 11].

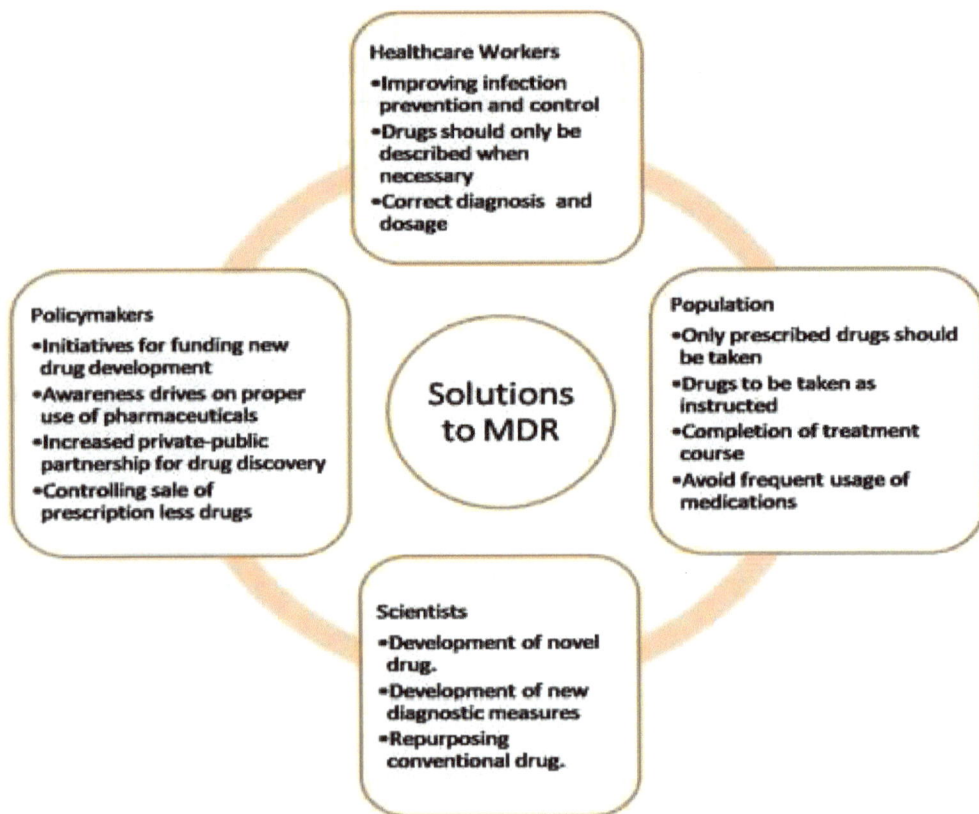

Fig. (2). Mitigation strategies for MDR.

Quinoline analogues, typically the newly synthesized triazine indole-quinoline hybrids, significantly inhibited the amastigotes and promastigotes of *L. donovani*. These compounds exhibited good antileishmanial profiles comparable to the standard drugs, pentamidine and miltefosine [12]. Excellent antimalarial success was achieved by a single compound from the porphyrin precursor series that has an IC_{50} value of 0.02μM, which is about 100 times lower than standard drug chloroquine (IC_{50} of 15 μM), thus can work at low dosage [13]. Novel scaffolds of symmetric terphenyl cyclic amidines showed better antimalarial potential than artemisinin and chloroquine [10]. Azadipeptide nitriles are another family of synthetics that are cogent inhibitors of falcipains (cysteine proteases responsible for haemoglobin degradation) in multidrug-resistant strains of *P. falciparum* [14].

The success of artemisinin probed the synthesis of novel synthetic derivatives of artemisinin such as 11-aza-artemisinin and dimers and trimers of the artemisinin hybrids. These showed brilliant activity against *Plasmodium falciparum* strains [15, 16]. A unique synthetic trioxolane, arterolane maleate in combination therapy with piperaquine, is under clinical trials, as a low cost effective oral drug for *P. falciparum* [17]. A series of hybrid 4-aminoquinolone 1,3,5-triazine derivatives revealed two compounds with IC_{50} values of 1-25 μM, inhibiting both chloroquine-sensitive and resistant *P. falciparum* strains [18].

Furthermore, a novel series of metronidazole-chalcone conjugates revealed two effective compounds against metronidazole (MTZ)-susceptible and MTZ-resistant protozoan strains [19]. A couple of nitrothiazole and benzothiazole derivatives showed excellent activity against *Trichomonas vaginalis* and *Giardia intestinalis* [20]. The chemical synthesis of uridine and adenosine analogues revealed a novel drug that remarkably controlled the cell growth of *T. vaginalis*. It is now US FDA approved for treating resistant trichomoniasis [21]. Disulfiram, an organic disulphide inactivated the *Giardia lamblia* kinase and the immunoreceptor tyrosine-based inhibition motif (ITIM). Thus, disulfiram is a prospective template for new pharmacotherapies against *G. Lamblia* [22].

DRUG DISCOVERY FROM NATURAL COMPOUND LIBRARIES

The development of low cost and validated drug targets is urgently needed to treat neglected protozoal diseases. Various scientists across the globe have been using *in-vitro* assays and bioinformatics to screen the natural biological products libraries in search of effective and safe antiprotozoal chemotherapies. The new chemical screenings can be broadly divided into protease and topoisomerase inhibitors and antimicrobial peptides [23].

Protease Inhibitors

Proteases are ubiquitous enzymes essential for many parasitic activities. Homologous proteases perform similar functions among the major pathogenic protists. It is thus an economically beneficial proposition to develop protease inhibitors against a wide variety of parasites. Cysteine protease (CP) inhibitors are one such class of drugs that can serve as broad-spectrum antiprotozoals [24, 25]. Leupeptin (derived from actinomycetes) and chymostatin (derived from streptomycetes) block cysteine proteases that facilitate the malarial parasite to cause rupture of host erythrocytes. These fungi derived molecules are further being used as scaffolds for the development of plasmodial proteases effective against both *P.falciparum* and *P.vivax* strains [26]. The derivatives of the epoxysuccinate peptide E64 extracted from *Aspergillus japonicum* are effective against cysteine proteases of the classes papain, cathepsin and calpain. This broad-spectrum protease inhibition activity makes E64 peptide quite effective against *Leishmania major, Entamoeba histolytica, Plasmodium spp.* and *Trypanosoma brucei strains* [27]. The endogenous CP inhibitor (ICP 1) of *E. histolytica* is another upcoming template for creating pharmaceuticals that modulate the function of CPs in amoebic lesions and reduce the adhesion of *E. histolytica* to extracellular matrix proteins [28].

Topoisomerase Inhibitors

DNA topoisomerases are omnipresent enzymes in the natural world responsible for DNA repair, replication, recombination and transcription processes. These are divided into ATP-independent (Type I) and ATP-dependent (Type II) enzymes [29]. The clinical success in anticancer therapy of the derivatives of a natural pentacyclic alkaloid, Camptothecin, extracted from the plant *Camptotheca accuminata*, marked topoisomerases as promising drug targets. It has been found that camptothecin is a potent inhibitor of topoisomerase type I of *P. falciparum, Leishmania spp.* and *Trypanosoma spp.* The suggested mechanism of this inhibitor is cellular apoptosis by launching a cascade of events initiated by blocking topoisomerase IB in the parasite cells. However, this molecule has heavy side effects and hence, its less toxic formulations, irinotecan and topotecan are now being explored for antiparasitic activity [30 - 33]. M-amsacrine and ofloxacin are topoisomerase II inhibitors that have displayed bioactivity against MDR *Trichomonas vaginalis* [34].

Antimicrobial Peptides

The innate immune response of the host releases antimicrobial peptides (AMPs) as the primary defence against pathogens. These are evolutionary conserved natural factors with anti-inflammatory and immunomodulation capacities. The two major advantages of utilising AMPs to tackle multidrug resistance is their swift pharmacokinetics and concentration-dependent non-receptor specific action that makes the selection of resistant strains unlikely [35, 36].

Dermaseptins, a type of AMP shows substantial activity against *P. falciparum, L. major, T.cruzi*. In addition, temporins and magainins are potential antimalarial and antileishmanial drugs. Although most AMPS are isolated from amphibian skin, mammalian AMPS also exist, which are produced by the skin and mucosal surfaces [35, 37]. Human salivary AMP, histatin 5 shows documented bioactivity against systemic parasitic protozoa by reducing ATP-synthesis in the pathogen. This AMP is a true cell-penetrating peptide and can be also be used as a drug delivery vector in addition to its chemotherapeutic uses [38]. The practical use of AMPs is restricted by their cost of production and large size. To circumvent this issue, the current thrust is in developing smaller synthetic peptidomimetics that mimic the mechanism of action of natural AMPs [39 - 41].

Other Natural Protozoa Inhibitors

Convolutamine occurs naturally in several plants and animals and is a highly effective antiparasitic compound, hindering the pathogenicity of trypanosomatids and nematodes [42]. Antigiardial and anti-amoebic activity were shown by two compounds, namely 3, 5- dicaffeoylquinic acid and sesquiterpene lactone produced by plants, *Artemisia argyi* and *Decachaeta incompta* respectively. Their derivatives are now being explored as novel drug targets for enhanced clearance of gastrointestinal and urinary tract pathogenic protozoa [43, 44]. Curcumin is a polyphenol produced by the plant *Curcuma longa* and a series of its analogues display *in-vitro* activity against *T. brucei* species and *P. falciparum*. The polypharmacology of curcumin enables a multifarious cascade of antiparasitic activities and hence, presents a low-resistance profile. This well-tolerated compound with negligible side effects is an excellent template for developing novel and safe antiprotozoals [45].

Another consideration in drug discovery is to reduce the toxic side effects of new drugs and for this, we should identify drug targets that are not present in humans. One such target is the sulphur assimilatory *de novo* L-cysteine biosynthetic pathway vital for several cellular activities of *E. histolytica*. Since the pathway is not present in humans, its pharmaceutical potential is worth exploring. Three natural compounds, xanthofulvin, pencolide and exophillic acid isolated from fungal broths were able to disrupt the cysteine synthase enzymes crucial for this pathway. These compounds present themselves as templates for safe anti-amoebic drugs to tackle metranidazole resistant *E. histolytica* infections [46, 47].

THE DRUG REPURPOSING APPROACH

The journey from drug discovery to commercial licensing is quite arduous. The last line of chemotherapies against protozoa are also falling prey to MDR and there is an urgent need for the introduction of new antiparasitics in clinical set-ups. The repurposing of licensed drugs is a valuable option, as these are already validated for their clinical use. This significantly reduces development costs as well.

Broad-spectrum antibiotics in combination therapies have effective antimalarial activity. Doxycycline in combination with quinidine and quinine is used as a treatment option for MDR *Plasmodium* species [48]. However, one should be careful to repurpose antibiotics due to the threat of the emergence of resistance to them or the existence of resistance in the clinical world. A good candidate for repurposing is the sulphonamide group, a key component in medicines to treat glaucoma, epilepsy and kidney disorders. The FDA approved sulphonamide, co-trimoxazole is being used as a treatment for pediatric malaria caused by *P. falciparum* [49].

Table 1. Highly effective novel drugs recently developed for MDR parasitic protozoa.

Major Parasitic Protozoan	MDR Profile	Novel Drug	Efficacy	References
Plasmodium falciparum	Chloroquine, artemisinin	Arterolane	Highly effective in combination with piperaquine	[17, 50]
Entamoeba histolytica	Metronidazole (MTZ), iodoquinol	Auranofin (repurposed rheumatoid arthritis drug)	10-fold greater activity than MTZ	[51]
Leishmania spp.	Pentavalent antimonials, miltefosine	Aminopyrazoles	High efficacy and immune to MDR pumps	[9]
Trypanosoma brucei, T.b. rhodesiense	Pentamidine, melarsoprol	Artemisinin derivatives and curcumin analogues	Low toxicity and high efficacy	[52, 53]

Paromomycin, an aminosidine antibiotic has recently been adapted to treat cutaneous leishmaniasis, giardiasis and amoebiasis [54, 55]. Research is ongoing to decode the exact antiprotozoal mechanism of paromomycin, to create derivatives that help reduce its MDR emergence potential. Artemisinin and its analogues show successful inhibition of *T. cruzi, T. b. rhodesiense,* and *Leishmania* species and are now being developed as alternatives to parasitic MDR kinetoplastids [52, 56].

High throughput screening of clinical drug libraries by the whole-cell-based method yielded hits for major parasitic protozoa. The rheumatoid arthritis drug auranofin exhibited ten-fold greater activity than the standard metranidazole (MTZ) against *E. histolytica* [51]. Some hits such as cycloheximide, doxorubicin hydrochloride, mitomycin C and other antineoplastic agents were inhibitory against three or more species of pathogenic protozoa and are now being further explored [57].

THERAPEUTIC APPLICATIONS OF RNA INTERFERENCE (RNAI)

Recent advances in RNAi technology have revealed the therapeutic application of small interfering RNAs (siRNAs) as antiparasitics by enabling direct inhibition of protozoa gene expression. The major limitation of this approach is the poor delivery of negatively charged nucleic acids inside cells. To overcome this limitation, very recently, a self-assembling β-glucan nanovector was developed that safely delivered the encapsulated siRNAs into the skin. Thus, this anti-inflammatory nanomedicine can deliver antiparasitic siRNAs directly to the sites of infection [58]. A wide variety of cell-penetrating peptides (CPPs) has been explored for the introduction of siRNAs into the human body. These are currently at preclinical levels. The CPP vehicle is rapid, biologically stable, lacks toxicity and displays chemotherapeutic potential [59]. The CPP, Transportan 10, a 21 amino acid peptide derived from wasp venom, is strongly bioactive against the blood stages of *P. falciparum* when coupled with primaquine [60].

Transmembrane kinases are considered potential drug targets for *E. histolytica* because of their role in virulence and proliferation. Abhyankar et.al showed that phagocytosis and endocytosis are downregulated by decreasing expression of the transmembrane kinase (*Eh*TMKB1-9). Hence, siRNA based gene silencing can be developed against these amoebic kinases [61, 62]. The increased expression of argininosuccinate synthetase (ARGG) in a drug-resistant strain of *L. infantum* is another target for siRNA mediated downregulation and control of MDR leishmaniasis [63].

COMPUTATIONAL–BASED STRATEGIES FOR DRUG DISCOVERY

It is crucial to employ a holistic approach to chemotherapeutic research. Computational and mathematical modelling of the complex interplay of host-parasite interactions under the systems biology branch of study helps in the discovery of potential drug targets. Using systems biology, the investigators have correctly predicted the targets of protozoal inhibitors by comparing models of chloroquine-resistant and chloroquine-sensitive *Plasmodium* genomes and analyzing the rewiring of parasitic genomes under drug pressure. This underpins the importance of computer-aided genomic tools in combination with growth inhibition assays to understand the MDR mechanism and identify novel drug scaffolds [62, 64].

Computational programmes have upgraded to improve the hit identification, hit-to-lead, and lead optimization stages of drug discovery, paving way for safer and better therapeutic molecules. As described above for screening natural and clinical drug libraries, one approach is the whole cell-based screening method [65]. Another technique gaining acceleration is *in-silico* profiling, which is the pre-screening of compound libraries to identify new chemical therapeutics for parasitic diseases. These approaches are relatively low cost as compared to the whole-library screening. Pre-screening along with molecular docking analyses helps in compound prioritization based on the mode of action, biochemistry and resistance data profiles. Sateriale *et al.* used protein sequences in a target-based screening method to examine libraries for potential bioactive compounds. This proteomic analysis of 13 parasite proteomes including *Plasmodium, Leishmania, and Trypanosoma* species, resulted in substantially higher hit rates in the pre-screened library in comparison to un-screened compounds [66]. The hits and the subsequent *in-silico* data of the hits have importance in the drug discovery and the drug repurposing studies. Furthermore, chemoinformatics tools utilised to comb through CRISPR arrayed libraries and compound databases to identify potential vaccine candidates and subsequent *in-silico* predictions of immunogenicity *via* B and T cell epitopes have renewed hopes for protozoa vaccine synthesis. Vaccine based prophylaxis is crucial for overcoming the emergence of new MDR strains [67].

CONCLUDING REMARKS

The multidrug resistance has seeped into treatment strategies for all parasitic protozoa. Additionally, even the last-resort drugs are showing signs of acquiring resistance. There is a dire need for mechanistically novel, safe and low-cost antiprotozoal drugs for use in clinical settings. The data on pathogenic protozoa collected over the last 50 years has aided in creating antiparasitics that are used throughout the world. This approach is being furthered with the data from genomic and metabolomics studies to create original drugs ranging from heterocyclic aromatics to quinoline and chalcone analogues. The computer-aided screening of natural compound libraries has revealed novel protease and topoisomerase inhibitors and antimicrobial peptides along with secondary metabolites from bacteria and fungi, which are significantly effective in controlling parasitic protozoa at better IC_{50} values than existing clinical therapies. This enables these new drugs to work at a low dosage and consequently present only low-grade side effects.

The rapid development of MDR protozoa particularly in developing countries, and the paucity of substantial research funding creates a vacuum in the discovery and approval of alternative antiprotozoal strategies Several such drugs are simply sitting in the pipeline, awaiting authorisation for commercial use. Drug repurposing to combat MDR is an intelligent and cost-effective way to fast-track this process because it reduces the time-lapse between drug discovery and clinical use. Antineoplastics, antitumor agents, broad-spectrum antibiotics and antifungals are commercially licensed drugs that are being explored for their potential to treat MDR parasitic protozoa. Advanced molecular techniques of siRNA mediated gene regulation to attack pathogenic capabilities of protozoa is an emerging field of therapeutics

To enable quicker licensing of effective drugs, investigative bodies are now shifting to a "non-inferiority" study design, in which the new chemotherapy is deemed acceptable if it performs "at least as well as" a currently approved therapy. This is essential to bring non-toxic and unique compounds into the market to fight the alarming rise of MDR protozoa. This chapter has provided a comprehensive account of the recent developments in therapeutics to circumvent the rising multidrug resistance in parasitic protozoa.

FUTURE PERSPECTIVE

Nearly a century of administering chemotherapy and the simultaneous development of drug resistance has taught us the most crucial lessons for effective disease control. Over-reliance on chemotherapy and careless prescription of drugs has contributed to the rapid rise in drug resistance. This century has concretized the dogma, prevention is better than cure, where insecticides for vector control and sanitization have managed protozoal diseases well by reducing transmission. It is observed that some drugs develop resistance faster than others and after the detailed analysis of drug-pathogen interplay, it was concluded that drugs with multiple targets (polypharmacology) have a lower resistance profile and thus, a lower chance of becoming ineffective [2]. Combinatorial therapies with synergistic actions are also quite beneficial. As seen with ACT (artemisinin combination therapy), the partner drugs clear the parasites that survive the short fatal exposure to artemisinin, keeping resistance at bay. However, it is wise to keep in mind that it can be risky to include a drug in a combination therapy after it has been reported ineffective because it may lead to failure of the partner drugs due to inefficient pathogen clearance [2].

The advancements in protozoa genome sequencing and the creation of drug discovery databases tailored to parasitic protozoa have greatly boosted the development of safer chemotherapies. Modern drug development is an expensive proposition and the lack of funding has subjected these diseases to severe neglect, despite affecting more than 500 million people worldwide [68]. The Drugs for Neglected Diseases *initiative* (DND*i*) organization, a successful R&D partnership, based in Geneva, Switzerland was founded in 2003 by seven institutions, including the Indian Council for Medical Research (ICMR). This is a welcome step in bridging the gap in the availability of effective and safe medicines targeting protozoa. To become future-ready when all existing conventional therapies become ineffective, the establishment of such public-private partnerships (PPPs) with a specific focus on tropical disease drug discovery is crucial.

CONSENT FOR PUBLICATION

Not applicable.

CONFLICT OF INTEREST

The authors declare no conflict of interest, financial or otherwise.

ACKNOWLEDGEMENTS

We extend our appreciation to the Amity University Rajasthan, Jaipur, India for its valuable support throughout the work.

REFERENCES

[1]   Tanwar J, Das S, Fatima Z, Hameed S. Multidrug resistance: an emerging crisis. Interdiscip Perspect Infect Dis 2014; 2014: 541340.

[2]   Koning HP, De . Drug resistance in protozoan parasites. Emerg Top Life Sci 2017; 1(6): 627-32.

[3]   Capela R, Moreira R, Lopes F. An overview of drug resistance in protozoal diseases. International Journal of Molecular Sciences. MDPI AG 2019; Vol. 20.

[4]   Kappagoda S, Singh U, Blackburn BG. Antiparasitic therapy. Mayo Clin Proc 2011; 86(6): 561-83.
[http://dx.doi.org/10.4065/mcp.2011.0203]

[5]   Monzote L, Siddiq A. Drug development to protozoan diseases. Open Med Chem J 2011; 5: 1-3.
[http://dx.doi.org/10.2174/1874104501105010001] [PMID: 21629506]

[6]   Agents A, Lee S, Kim M, Hayat F, Shin D. Recent advances in the discovery of novel antiprotozoal agents. Molecules 2019; 24(21): 3886.

[7]   Plano D, Baquedano Y, Moreno-Mateos D, *et al.* Selenocyanates and diselenides: a new class of potent antileishmanial agents. Eur J Med Chem 2011; 46(8): 3315-23.
[http://dx.doi.org/10.1016/j.ejmech.2011.04.054] [PMID: 21571403]

[8]   Rashid U, Sultana R, Shaheen N, *et al.* Structure based medicinal chemistry-driven strategy to design substituted dihydropyrimidines as potential antileishmanial agents. Eur J Med Chem 2016; 115: 230-44.
[http://dx.doi.org/10.1016/j.ejmech.2016.03.022] [PMID: 27017551]

[9]   Van den Kerkhof M, Mabille D, Hendrickx S, *et al.* Antileishmanial aminopyrazoles: Studies into mechanisms and stability of experimental drug resistance. Antimicrob Agents Chemother 2020; 64(9): e00152-20.
[http://dx.doi.org/10.1128/AAC.00152-20] [PMID: 32601168]

[10]   Patrick DA, Ismail MA, Arafa RK, *et al.* Synthesis and antiprotozoal activity of dicationic m-terphenyl and 1,3-dipyridylbenzene derivatives. J Med Chem 2013; 56(13): 5473-94.
[http://dx.doi.org/10.1021/jm400508e] [PMID: 23795673]

[11]   Trunz BB, Jędrysiak R, Tweats D, *et al.* 1-Aryl-4-nitro-1H-imidazoles, a new promising series for the treatment of human African trypanosomiasis. Eur J Med Chem 2011; 46(5): 1524-35.
[http://dx.doi.org/10.1016/j.ejmech.2011.01.071] [PMID: 21353728]

[12]   Sharma R, Pandey AK, Shivahare R, Srivastava K, Gupta S, Chauhan PMS. Triazino indole-quinoline hybrid: a novel approach to antileishmanial agents. Bioorg Med Chem Lett 2014; 24(1): 298-301.
[http://dx.doi.org/10.1016/j.bmcl.2013.11.018] [PMID: 24314395]

[13]   Abada Z, Cojean S, Pomel S, *et al.* Synthesis and antiprotozoal activity of original porphyrin precursors and derivatives. Eur J Med Chem 2013; 67: 158-65.
[http://dx.doi.org/10.1016/j.ejmech.2013.06.002] [PMID: 23851117]

[14]   Löser R, Gut J, Rosenthal PJ, Frizler M, Gütschow M, Andrews KT. Antimalarial activity of azadipeptide nitriles. Bioorg Med Chem Lett 2010; 20(1): 252-5.

[http://dx.doi.org/10.1016/j.bmcl.2009.10.122] [PMID: 19913414]

[15]   Nguyen Le T, De Borggraeve WM, Grellier P, Pham VC, Dehaen W, Nguyen VH. Synthesis of 11-aza-artemisinin derivatives using the Ugi reaction and an evaluation of their antimalarial activity. Tetrahedron Lett 2014; 55(35): 4892-4.
[http://dx.doi.org/10.1016/j.tetlet.2014.07.027]

[16]   Reiter C, Fröhlich T, Gruber L, *et al.* Highly potent artemisinin-derived dimers and trimers: Synthesis and evaluation of their antimalarial, antileukemia and antiviral activities. Bioorg Med Chem 2015; 23(17): 5452-8.
[http://dx.doi.org/10.1016/j.bmc.2015.07.048] [PMID: 26260339]

[17]   Toure OA, Rulisa S, Anvikar AR, *et al.* Efficacy and safety of fixed dose combination of arterolane maleate and piperaquine phosphate dispersible tablets in paediatric patients with acute uncomplicated Plasmodium falciparum malaria: a phase II, multicentric, open-label study. Malar J 2015; 14(1): 469.
[http://dx.doi.org/10.1186/s12936-015-0982-y] [PMID: 26608469]

[18]   Bhat HR, Singh UP, Thakur A, *et al.* Synthesis, antimalarial activity and molecular docking of hybrid 4-aminoquinoline-1,3,5-triazine derivatives. Exp Parasitol 2015; 157: 59-67.
[http://dx.doi.org/10.1016/j.exppara.2015.06.016] [PMID: 26164360]

[19]   Anthwal A, Rajesh UC, Rawat MSM, *et al.* Novel metronidazole-chalcone conjugates with potential to counter drug resistance in Trichomonas vaginalis. Eur J Med Chem 2014; 79: 89-94.
[http://dx.doi.org/10.1016/j.ejmech.2014.03.076] [PMID: 24727243]

[20]   Navarrete-Vázquez G, Chávez-Silva F, Colín-Lozano B, *et al.* Synthesis of nitro(benzo)thiazole acetamides and in vitro antiprotozoal effect against amitochondriate parasites Giardia intestinalis and Trichomonas vaginalis. Bioorg Med Chem 2015; 23(9): 2204-10.
[http://dx.doi.org/10.1016/j.bmc.2015.02.059] [PMID: 25801157]

[21]   Shokar A, Au A, An SH, *et al.* S-Adenosylhomocysteine hydrolase of the protozoan parasite Trichomonas vaginalis: potent inhibitory activity of 9-(2-deoxy-2-fluoro-β,D-arabinofuranosyl) adenine. Bioorg Med Chem Lett 2012; 22(12): 4203-5.
[http://dx.doi.org/10.1016/j.bmcl.2012.03.087] [PMID: 22579483]

[22]   Castillo-Villanueva A, Rufino-González Y, Méndez ST, *et al.* Disulfiram as a novel inactivator of Giardia lamblia triosephosphate isomerase with antigiardial potential. Int J Parasitol Drugs Drug Resist 2017; 7(3): 425-32.
[http://dx.doi.org/10.1016/j.ijpddr.2017.11.003] [PMID: 29197728]

[23]   Zucca M, Savoia D. Current developments in the therapy of protozoan infections. Open Med Chem J 2011; 5: 4-10.
[http://dx.doi.org/10.2174/1874104501105010004] [PMID: 21629507]

[24]   Rascón AA Jr, McKerrow JH. Synthetic and natural protease inhibitors provide insights into parasite development, virulence and pathogenesis. Curr Med Chem 2013; 20(25): 3078-102.
[http://dx.doi.org/10.2174/0929867311320250005] [PMID: 23514418]

[25]   Siqueira-Neto JL, Debnath A, McCall LI, Bernatchez JA, Ndao M, Reed SL, *et al.* Cysteine proteases in protozoan parasites. PLOS. 2018.
[http://dx.doi.org/10.1371/journal.pntd.0006512]

[26]   Vidal-Albalat A, González FV. Natural Products as Cathepsin Inhibitors. Studies in Natural Products Chemistry. Elsevier B.V. 2016; pp. 179-213.

[27]   Siklos M, BenAissa M, Thatcher GRJ. Cysteine proteases as therapeutic targets: Does selectivity matter? A systematic review of calpain and cathepsin inhibitors. Vol. 5, Acta Pharmaceutica Sinica B. Chinese Academy of Medical Sciences. 2015; pp. 506-19.

[28]   Lee YA, Saito-Nakano Y, Kim KA, Min A, Nozaki T, Shin MH. Modulation of endogenous Cysteine Protease Inhibitor (ICP) 1 expression in Entamoeba histolytica affects amoebic adhesion to Extracellular Matrix proteins. Exp Parasitol 2015; 149: 7-15.

[http://dx.doi.org/10.1016/j.exppara.2014.12.001] [PMID: 25500214]

[29] Reguera RM, Díaz-González R, Pérez-Pertejo Y, Balaña-Fouce R. Characterizing the bi-subunit type IB DNA topoisomerase of Leishmania parasites; a novel scenario for drug intervention in trypanosomatids. Curr Drug Targets 2008; 9(11): 966-78.
[http://dx.doi.org/10.2174/138945008786786118] [PMID: 18991609]

[30] Zuma AA, Mendes IC, Reignault LC, *et al.* How Trypanosoma cruzi handles cell cycle arrest promoted by camptothecin, a topoisomerase I inhibitor. Mol Biochem Parasitol 2014; 193(2): 93-100.
[http://dx.doi.org/10.1016/j.molbiopara.2014.02.001] [PMID: 24530483]

[31] Prada CF, Álvarez-Velilla R, Balaña-Fouce R, *et al.* Gimatecan and other camptothecin derivatives poison Leishmania DNA-topoisomerase IB leading to a strong leishmanicidal effect. Biochem Pharmacol 2013; 85(10): 1433-40.
[http://dx.doi.org/10.1016/j.bcp.2013.02.024] [PMID: 23466420]

[32] Sen N, Das BB, Ganguly A, *et al.* Camptothecin induced mitochondrial dysfunction leading to programmed cell death in unicellular hemoflagellate Leishmania donovani. Cell Death Differ 2004; 11(8): 924-36.
[http://dx.doi.org/10.1038/sj.cdd.4401435] [PMID: 15118764]

[33] Deterding A, Dungey FA, Thompson KA, Steverding D. Anti-trypanosomal activities of DNA topoisomerase inhibitors. Acta Trop 2005; 93(3): 311-6.
[http://dx.doi.org/10.1016/j.actatropica.2005.01.005] [PMID: 15715983]

[34] Sithiprom S, Petmitr S C-PP. Partial purification and characterization of Trichomonas vaginalis DNA topoisomerase II. Southeast Asian J Trop Med Public Heal 2009; 40(5): 877-5.

[35] Rivas L, Luque-Ortega JR, Andreu D. Amphibian antimicrobial peptides and Protozoa: lessons from parasites. Biochim Biophys Acta 2009; 1788(8): 1570-81.
[http://dx.doi.org/10.1016/j.bbamem.2008.11.002] [PMID: 19046939]

[36] Steinstraesser L, Kraneburg UM, Hirsch T, *et al.* Host defense peptides as effector molecules of the innate immune response: a sledgehammer for drug resistance? Int J Mol Sci 2009; 10(9): 3951-70.
[http://dx.doi.org/10.3390/ijms10093951] [PMID: 19865528]

[37] Savoia D, Guerrini R, Marzola E, Salvadori S. Synthesis and antimicrobial activity of dermaseptin S1 analogues. Bioorg Med Chem 2008; 16(17): 8205-9.
[http://dx.doi.org/10.1016/j.bmc.2008.07.032] [PMID: 18676150]

[38] Luque-Ortega JR, van't Hof W, Veerman ECI, Saugar JM, Rivas L. Human antimicrobial peptide histatin 5 is a cell-penetrating peptide targeting mitochondrial ATP synthesis in Leishmania. FASEB J 2008; 22(6): 1817-28.
[http://dx.doi.org/10.1096/fj.07-096081] [PMID: 18230684]

[39] Saviello MR, Malfi S, Campiglia P, *et al.* New insight into the mechanism of action of the temporin antimicrobial peptides. Biochemistry 2010; 49(7): 1477-85.
[http://dx.doi.org/10.1021/bi902166d] [PMID: 20082523]

[40] Sharma RK, Reddy RP, Tegge W, Jain R. Discovery of Trp-His and His-Arg analogues as new structural classes of short antimicrobial peptides. J Med Chem 2009; 52(23): 7421-31.
[http://dx.doi.org/10.1021/jm900622d] [PMID: 19655779]

[41] Rodziewicz-Motowidło S, Mickiewicz B, Greber K, *et al.* Antimicrobial and conformational studies of the active and inactive analogues of the protegrin-1 peptide. FEBS J 2010; 277(4): 1010-22.
[http://dx.doi.org/10.1111/j.1742-4658.2009.07544.x] [PMID: 20074208]

[42] Pham NB, Deydier S, Labaied M, Monnerat S, Stuart K, Quinn RJ. N^1,N^1-Dimethyl-N^3-(--(trifluoromethyl)phenethyl)propane-1,3-diamine, a new lead for the treatment of human African trypanosomiasis. Eur J Med Chem 2014; 74: 541-51.
[http://dx.doi.org/10.1016/j.ejmech.2013.12.050] [PMID: 24530464]

[43] Bautista E, Calzada F, Yepez-Mulia L, Chavez-Soto M, Ortega A. Incomptines C and D, two

heliangolides from Decachaeta incompta and their antiprotozoal activity. Planta Med 2012; 78(15): 1698-701.
[http://dx.doi.org/10.1055/s-0032-1315255] [PMID: 22948610]

[44]   Zhang YH, Xue MQ, Bai YC, Yuan HH, Zhao HL, Lan MB. 3,5-Dicaffeoylquinic acid isolated from Artemisia argyi and its ester derivatives exert anti-leucyl-tRNA synthetase of Giardia lamblia (GlLeuRS) and potential anti-giardial effects. Fitoterapia 2012; 83(7): 1281-5.
[http://dx.doi.org/10.1016/j.fitote.2012.05.016] [PMID: 22668973]

[45]   Chakrabarti R, Rawat PS, Cooke BM, Coppel RL, Patankar S. Cellular Effects of Curcumin on Plasmodium falciparum Include Disruption of Microtubules. PLoS One. 2013; 8: p. (3)e57302.
[http://dx.doi.org/10.1371/journal.pone.0057302]

[46]   Mori M, Tsuge S, Fukasawa W, *et al.* Discovery of antiamebic compounds that inhibit cysteine synthase from the enteric parasitic protist *entamoeba histolytica* by screening of microbial secondary metabolites. Front Cell Infect Microbiol 2018; 8: 409.
[http://dx.doi.org/10.3389/fcimb.2018.00409] [PMID: 30568921]

[47]   Mori M, Jeelani G, Masuda Y, *et al.* Identification of natural inhibitors of Entamoeba histolytica cysteine synthase from microbial secondary metabolites. Front Microbiol 2015; 6(SEP): 962.
[http://dx.doi.org/10.3389/fmicb.2015.00962] [PMID: 26441896]

[48]   Tan KR, Magill AJ, Parise ME, Arguin PM. Doxycycline for malaria chemoprophylaxis and treatment: Report from the CDC expert meeting on malaria chemoprophylaxis. American Journal of Tropical Medicine and Hygiene. The American Society of Tropical Medicine and Hygiene 2011; pp. 517-31.
[http://dx.doi.org/10.4269/ajtmh.2011.10-0285]

[49]   Manyando C, Njunju EM, D'Alessandro U, Van geertruyden J-P. Van geertruyden JP. Safety and Efficacy of Co-Trimoxazole for Treatment and Prevention of *Plasmodium falciparum* Malaria: A Systematic Review. Vol. 8, PLoS ONE. PLoS One 2013; 8(2): e56916.
[http://dx.doi.org/10.1371/journal.pone.0056916]

[50]   Valecha N, Looareesuwan S, Martensson A, *et al.* Arterolane, a new synthetic trioxolane for treatment of uncomplicated Plasmodium falciparum malaria: a phase II, multicenter, randomized, dose-finding clinical trial. Clin Infect Dis 2010; 51(6): 684-91.
[http://dx.doi.org/10.1086/655831] [PMID: 20687837]

[51]   Debnath A, Parsonage D, Andrade RM, *et al.* A high-throughput drug screen for Entamoeba histolytica identifies a new lead and target. Nat Med 2012; 18(6): 956-60.
[http://dx.doi.org/10.1038/nm.2758] [PMID: 22610278]

[52]   Loo CSN, Lam NSK, Yu D. Artemisinin and its derivatives in treating protozoan infections beyond malaria. Pharmacological Research. Academic Press 2017; 117: pp. 192-217.

[53]   Ettari R, Previti S, Maiorana S, *et al.* Drug combination studies of curcumin and genistein against rhodesain of *Trypanosoma brucei rhodesiense*. Nat Prod Res 2019; 33(24): 3577-81.
[http://dx.doi.org/10.1080/14786419.2018.1483927] [PMID: 29897253]

[54]   Davidson RN, den Boer M, Ritmeijer K. Paromomycin. Trans R Soc Trop Med Hyg 2009; 103(7): 653-60.
[http://dx.doi.org/10.1016/j.trstmh.2008.09.008] [PMID: 18947845]

[55]   Ben Salah A, Ben Messaoud N, Guedri E, *et al.* Topical paromomycin with or without gentamicin for cutaneous leishmaniasis. N Engl J Med 2013; 368(6): 524-32.
[http://dx.doi.org/10.1056/NEJMoa1202657] [PMID: 23388004]

[56]   Sen R, Ganguly S, Saha P, Chatterjee M. Efficacy of artemisinin in experimental visceral leishmaniasis. Int J Antimicrob Agents 2010; 36(1): 43-9.
[http://dx.doi.org/10.1016/j.ijantimicag.2010.03.008] [PMID: 20403680]

[57]   Andrews KT, Fisher G, Skinner-Adams TS. Drug repurposing and human parasitic protozoan diseases.

Int J Parasitol Drugs Drug Resist 2014; 4(2): 95-111.
[http://dx.doi.org/10.1016/j.ijpddr.2014.02.002] [PMID: 25057459]

[58]   Lee K, Min D, Choi Y, *et al.* Self-Assembling β-Glucan Nanomedicine for the Delivery of siRNA. Biomedicines 2020; 8(11): 1-11.
[http://dx.doi.org/10.3390/biomedicines8110497] [PMID: 33198404]

[59]   Keller AA, Scheiding B, Breitling R, *et al.* Transduction and transfection of difficult-to-transfect cells: Systematic attempts for the transfection of protozoa Leishmania. J Cell Biochem 2019; 120(1): 14-27.
[http://dx.doi.org/10.1002/jcb.27463] [PMID: 30216507]

[60]   Aguiar L, Biosca A, Lantero E, *et al.* Coupling the antimalarial cell penetrating peptide TP10 to classical antimalarial drugs primaquine and chloroquine produces strongly hemolytic conjugates. Molecules 2019; 24(24): E4559.
[http://dx.doi.org/10.3390/molecules24244559] [PMID: 31842498]

[61]   Abhyankar MM, Shrimal S, Gilchrist CA, Bhattacharya A, Petri WA Jr. The Entamoeba histolytica serum-inducible transmembrane kinase EhTMKB1-9 is involved in intestinal amebiasis. Int J Parasitol Drugs Drug Resist 2012; 2: 243-8.
[http://dx.doi.org/10.1016/j.ijpddr.2012.01.002] [PMID: 23267432]

[62]   Buckner FS, Waters NC, Avery VM. Recent highlights in anti-protozoan drug development and resistance research. Int J Parasitol Drugs Drug Resist 2012; 2: 230-5.
[http://dx.doi.org/10.1016/j.ijpddr.2012.05.002] [PMID: 24533285]

[63]   El Fadili K, Drummelsmith J, Roy G, Jardim A, Ouellette M. Down regulation of KMP-11 in Leishmania infantum axenic antimony resistant amastigotes as revealed by a proteomic screen. Exp Parasitol 2009; 123(1): 51-7.
[http://dx.doi.org/10.1016/j.exppara.2009.05.013] [PMID: 19500579]

[64]   Pradhan A, Siwo GH, Singh N, *et al.* Chemogenomic profiling of Plasmodium falciparum as a tool to aid antimalarial drug discovery. Sci Rep 2015; 5: 15930.
[http://dx.doi.org/10.1038/srep15930] [PMID: 26541648]

[65]   Njogu PM, Guantai EM, Pavadai E, Chibale K. Computer-Aided drug discovery approaches against the tropical infectious diseases malaria, tuberculosis, trypanosomiasis, and leishmaniasis. ACS Infectious Diseases American Chemical Society. 2016; 2: pp. 8-31.

[66]   Sateriale A, Bessoff K, Sarkar IN, Huston CD. Drug repurposing: mining protozoan proteomes for targets of known bioactive compounds. J Am Med Inform Assoc 2014; 21(2): 238-44.
[http://dx.doi.org/10.1136/amiajnl-2013-001700] [PMID: 23757409]

[67]   Gómez Marín JE, El Bissati K. Editorial: Innovative Therapeutic and Immunomodulatory Strategies for Protozoan Infections. Frontiers in Cellular and Infection Microbiology. Frontiers Media S.A. 2019; Vol. 9: p. 293.

[68]   Naghavi M, Wang H, Lozano R, Davis A, Liang X, Zhou M, *et al.* Global, regional, and national age-sex specific all-cause and cause-specific mortality for 240 causes of death, 1990-2013: a systematic analysis for the Global Burden of Disease Study 2013. Lancet 2015; 385(9963): 117-71.
[http://dx.doi.org/10.1016/S0140-6736(14)61682-2] [PMID: 25530442]

SUBJECT INDEX

A